D1477791

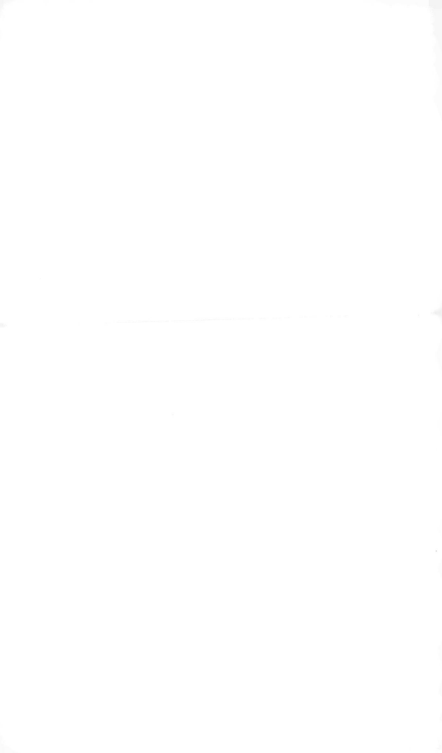

CELIA ROBERTS
ADRIAN MACKENZIE
MAGGIE MORT

with
THERESA ATKINSON
METTE KRAGH-FURBO
JOANN WILKINSON

LIVING DATA

Making Sense of Health Biosensing

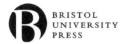

BRISTOL
UNIVERSITY
PRESS

First published in Great Britain in 2019 by

Bristol University Press
University of Bristol
1-9 Old Park Hill
Bristol
BS2 8BB
UK
t: +44 (0)117 954 5940
www.bristoluniversitypress.co.uk

North America office:
Bristol University Press
c/o The University of Chicago Press
1427 East 60th Street
Chicago, IL 60637, USA
t: +1 773 702 7700
f: +1 773 702 9756
sales@press.uchicago.edu
www.press.uchicago.edu

© Bristol University Press 2019

British Library Cataloguing in Publication Data
A catalogue record for this book is available from the British Library.

Library of Congress Cataloging-in-Publication Data
A catalog record for this book has been requested.

ISBN 978-1-5292-0750-7 (hardback)
ISBN 978-1-5292-0753-8 (ePub)
ISBN 978-1-5292-0751-4 (ePDF)

The right of Celia Roberts, Adrian Mackenzie and Maggie Mort to be identified as authors of this
work has been asserted by them in accordance with the Copyright, Designs and Patents Act 1988.

Cover design by blu inc, Bristol
Front cover: image kindly supplied by Shutterstock
Printed and bound in Great Britain by CPI Group (UK) Ltd,
Croydon, CR0 4YY
Bristol University Press uses environmentally responsible print
partners

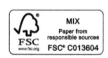

Contents

List of Tables, Figures and Boxes

Acknowledgements

First we would like to thank all the respondents to our different research projects drawn on in this book who for reasons of confidentiality must remain anonymous, as must the members of the citizens' panels we convened for the EFORTT project with the support of the European Commission's FP7 Science in Society Programme (no 217787).

The role and influence of anthropologist Dawn Nafus has been pivotal to our work on biosensing. Her intellectual curiosity, generosity and political engagement are inspiring. We acknowledge the support of Intel's University Research Office which funded the Biosensors in Everyday Life programme, the two associated doctoral projects and one of our citizens' panels. It was immensely rewarding for all members of our group to meet with Intel researchers at their offices in the US and Ireland, in particular David Prendergast. We must also thank our fellow researchers on that programme for many thought-provoking discussions: Nina Wakeford, Celia Lury, Sophie Day, Mark Böhlen, Gina Neff and Britany Fiore-Gartland.

Further support for doctoral research into telecare was provided by the Economic and Social Research Council's Northwest Doctoral Training Programme, and the ethnographic work was also supported by a Local Authority. We are particularly grateful for the support of our European project colleagues, Christine Milligan, Daniel Lopez Gomez, Miguel Domenech, Blanca Callén, Tomás Sánchez Criado, Ingunn Moser, Hilde Thygesen, Dick Willems, Jeannette Pols, Josie Baxter and Craig Frost, and also Elham Kashefi and Louis Neven, for their intellectual and practical help in supporting this work. We would also like to thank Brigit McWade and Oscar Javier Maldonado Castañeda, who provided research assistance for the stress sensing chapter, and Sue Weldon for preparation and co-facilitation of the 'Our Bodies, Our Data' citizens' panel.

We are indebted to Cron Cronshaw for his careful and painstaking editorial assistance with this book. The views expressed here are the sole responsibility of the authors and do not necessarily reflect the views of the European Commission, Intel or the Economic and Social Research Council. It is important to note that ethical approval for the empirical work undertaken here was granted by the Faculty of Arts and Social Sciences Research Ethics Committee, Lancaster University.

Preface

In October 2010, Celia, Adrian and Maggie met in the Sociology Department coffee room at Lancaster University to discuss what to do after Celia had received a rather unusual email. The message was from 'Intel Labs', not an organisation that we had heard of, although, of course, we knew about the Intel Corporation. It contained a call for proposals for a three-year research programme called 'Biosensors in Everyday Life'; it seemed that Intel Labs wanted to know more about the possible uses and usabilities of what appeared to be a revolutionary new trend in the approach of 'middle-class users' to acquiring health-related knowledge about their bodies.

None of us had ever had research funding from a commercial technology company before and the programme was intriguing for us as researchers in the Science and Technology Studies field. Celia and Maggie had just finished working on a European study of 'remote-care' technologies and Adrian had been working on the data-intensive transformations of genomics. Celia's background in feminist studies of reproduction, sexuality and biomedicine, Adrian's in philosophy of technology and software studies, and Maggie's in technological change in health care and forms of public engagement and participation, all seemed to tell us that we should make a response to the approach from Intel Labs.

We decided to propose a project that would push at what seemed to be Intel's primary interest in middle-class users by opening up questions around two areas of contemporary social concern – infertility/conception and personal genetic testing – for which we offered to supervise two doctoral studies. To this, we added a third element: a parallel cross-cutting initiative to try to understand the public's (in addition to middle-class users') views about these developments. We thought that if the proposal gained favour with Intel Labs, then the research would be worthwhile and, we hoped, socially useful. If not, little would be lost.

In the event, we formed a productive and educative relationship with Intel Labs, and discovered that it employed talented and critical anthropologists with whom we went on to have great discussions. Our initial fears about corporate influence over our work proved unfounded, and at Lancaster, we decided to form the Living Data Research Group (see: www.livingdata. wordpress.com/about-us/) as our group expanded to include Mette Kragh-Furbo and Joann Wilkinson undertaking their PhD studies.

This book builds on the work we carried out for the Biosensors in Everyday Life programme: ethnographic studies of direct-to-consumer genetic testing and fertility monitoring; and a citizens' panel to deliberate on the findings of these and consider biosensing in society more broadly.[1] At the time, there was only sparse social-scientific work on fertility monitoring and very little discussion of this and direct-to-consumer genetic testing in public forums. We also discuss our earlier research on forms of 'telecare' undertaken for the European Commission's Framework 7 programme, together with material from a current, third doctoral study of remote-care system implementation, sponsored by the Economic and Social Research Council and undertaken by Theresa Atkinson. Finally, we have added a new topic – stress biosensing – which grew from Celia's and Adrian's interests in the neuroscience of parenting and was supported in its early stages by an additional small grant from Intel Labs.

Readers will note that the book's chapters follow the 'life course' in that they consider roles for biosensors in conception, childhood stress, monitoring adult risk and old-age care. We are looking at biosensors across the life course not so much in order to contribute to life-course literature, but because (and

---

[1]   The Appendix contains the narrative we used to frame the citizens' panel.

this links with our original proposal to Intel) we want to focus on a set of lived social problems (infertility, stress, genetic risk and social isolation in ageing) within which biosensors are projected to play a role, rather than on the classic 'quantified self' 30-something-year-old 'middle-class' constituency. In so doing, we also document biosensing's role in reshaping cultural conceptions and lived experiences of 'the (healthy) life course': marking the beginning and ends of 'the reproductive years'; refiguring intergenerational bodily connections; and changing what it means to be 'aged'.

Our title, *Living Data*, carries at least two meanings: that data is lived with, and in, by individuals, groups and constituencies; and that it is living, changing and proliferating in sometimes unpredictable ways. Our approach is critical, as will become clear, but we also argue that framing biosensing as a simple colonisation of bodies or an elaborate exercise in neoliberal self-governance is a rather limiting approach that fails to recognise either the strong attachments of individuals and groups to related practices and devices, or the more radical potential that biosensing may have for health and life projects.

Introduction: What Does Biosensing Do?

You would think that it would be obvious, but it is not: what is a biosensor? Biosensors have been defined by Intel anthropologist Dawn Nafus (2016a: xiii) as devices that 'indicate something about the body or the physical environment', and biosensing as a practice that 'uses information technology to understand something about bodies or the environment in which they live, whether the technology is at the cutting edge or not'. Standing at the intersection of everyday experience, scientific, medical and technical knowledges, media-platform economies, transformations in the biopolitics of health care, and cultural-material imaginaries of digital health, it is hardly surprising that biosensors are lively assemblages. They increasingly form a stage – a platform – on which problems of childhood, puberty, sexualities, reproduction, wellness, fitness, disease, ageing, medical expertise, health-care provision, economic productivity and citizenship, among others, play out.

Questions teem around these broad, pragmatic definitions of biosensors and biosensing. Are biosensors really concerned with 'the body' or 'the physical environment', or are they an outgrowth of the fitness and health-lifestyle industries? (Given that things seem to get inside us, do bodies live in an environment anyway?) Do the ideas of 'indicating' and 'understanding' accommodate what people do with biosensors? What else do they do with them? Do biosensors and biosensing challenge or extend traditional medical authority? Does biosensing increase people's control over their health, as is often claimed? What is the connection between more data and health? Who is biosensing who? What is the relation between biosensing and people's anxiety about their health? How do people subvert or reinvent biosensors to assure themselves of health? How does biosensing participate in making certain forms of selfhood and group viable? What socio-material networks do biosensing practices produce and rely on? Who is profiting from biosensing and who is not, and how? What new forms of work and care are produced in biosensing? How does the dream of continuous monitoring animate biosensing? How might collectives or communities thrive through biosensing? What, if any, policy framework might meet public concerns about health biosensors?

In this book, we offer some ways of responding to this panoply of questions and perhaps framing some new ones. We discuss a range of biosensors and biosensings, testing the boundaries of the technical definitions of biosensor in order to access emerging configurations and experiences that we consider relevant. Our approach to biosensing practices centres on contrasts between different biosensors and biosensing practices broadly concerned with health.

Table 0.1 suggests something of the gamut of biosensing practices and the range of understandings that might develop from them. The columns lay out a range of types of biosensing practice and correspond to contrasting approaches to health. Fitness, self-monitoring, clinical medicine, social care and environmental biosensing practices all relate to health. What is health? The absence of disease or illness? This definition will not do. It is a definition by negation, as in 'woman is the absence of man'. A concept of health needs positive and diverse content. The World Health Organisation definition from 1946 (WHO, 2006) is often quoted: 'Health is a state of complete physical, mental and social well-being and not merely the absence of disease or infirmity'. Another more puzzling definition, less anchored in absence, comes from the philosopher of medicine George Canguilhem (1989: 190), who sees health as 'the regulatory flywheel of the possibilities of reaction'. Canguilhem, writing in the mid-20th century, conjures up a slightly steampunk image of a spinning wheel storing up energy, and evening out

Table 0.1: Some biosensor domains and their dimensions

	Fitness	Self-health	Biomedical	Social care	Environmental
What is measured?	steps, cycling	sleeping, stress	genetic risk, blood sugar, weight	falls, enuresis	air, water, mercury
What are users supposed to do?	count, do more, do less	map, chart, analysis	test, monitor, contribute data, access clinics	accept monitoring, trigger care	count, record, aggregate
Devices and platforms	wearable, social media	wearable, social media	lab instrument, social media	wearable, fixed sensors, call centre	fixed sensor, apps
Role of groups	optional, competition	optional, comparison, social group	population, cohort	client/customer service, relatives	community group, social movement
Institutional proximity	low	low	medium	high	medium
Relevant knowledges	sport science, exercise physiology, military	psychology, women's health movement, military	life sciences, genomics, reproductive medicine	gerontology, physiology, health economics, public health	ecology, toxicology, hydrology

the flow of energy in an engine. Put in less engineered images, health is the capacity to bounce back from, recover from or adapt to altered conditions, including those associated with illness and disability. Biosensing practices engage with health in different ways, depart from different experiences, situations and knowledges of bodies, and yield different institutional, material and discursive arrangements. Whether and how they spin the regulatory flywheel is moot. They do pluralise health. The health of a fitness programme differs from the health of an environmental campaign for clean air; the health of continuous blood sugar monitoring for diabetes management differs from the monitoring of ovulation to maximise chances of conception, and so on. They configure and sometimes define individual and group identities. Given many healths, or many constructions of health for bodies, biosensing practices multiply.

Although we do not devote a chapter to each column of the table, the central columns of the table are the focus of the chapters: self-health, biomedical and social care biosensing (we have not conducted research on environmental biosensing, but excellent existing work in this field includes Tironi and Rodríguez Giralt [2017] and Pritchard, Gabrys and Houston [2018]). The five main biosensing practices we discuss – fertility monitoring, stress biosensing, DNA genotyping and falls monitoring – span times and places, life stages, forms of sensor and data, practices of interpreting and understanding, modes of practical organisation, and knowledge and expertise. In our analysis of these significantly different cases, we attend to the irreducible slippages and misalignments that arise when biosensing operates amid cultures and communities differently affected by institutional, state, corporate and political agencies. We want to make sense of areas of health – fertility, stress, susceptibilities and ageing – that concern people's sense of self, their sense of individual and collective agency, and their capacity to practically engage with the problems and potentials of their health.

Each of the biosensing practices that we explore has power-laden regulatory, economic and epistemic facets, sometimes reaching deep into the institutions and experiences of gender, kinship, ageing, citizenship and ethnicity. Each has deep temporal structures within life-worlds. Each permeates embodied senses of selfhood and relationality. Falls detectors, ovulation monitors, heart-rate monitors, cortisol tests and DNA genotyping have very different ways of dealing with bodies in time and the temporal structuring of life. The devices produce different kinds of data: micro-second time-stamped acceleration measurements; a series of time- and date-stamped temperature readings; a chemical concentration measurement (possibly date-stamped); and a list of half-a-million or more DNA variants without any obvious time or date stamp, but indirectly referring to patterns of heredity sometimes spanning geological epochs. Much of this data offers little immediate purchase for biological knowledge, let alone clinical intervention in any strict sense. Much of the data cannot be understood apart from individual medical histories, family history, patterns of everyday life and a whole habitus that renders them potentially meaningful. Our focus on stress, fertility, ageing and genetic susceptibility highlights both the times and bodies on different scales, ranging from the molecular (or even sub-molecular in the case of DNA variations), through cells (oocytes), to bodies across generations.

It may or may not be possible to locate all biosensing practices in Table 0.1. Either way, the point is to suggest diagrammatically the variety of positions opened up by biosensing, both in relation to the settled landscapes of biomedical practices and in relation to the transverse relationalities that could emerge. Does a self-health platform where people exchange, correlate and interpret exercise-related data afford the interventions, techniques of self or subjectivity that change the relation of self to self? Does the proximity of social care to state or civil society organisations such as social services or charities alter when telecare monitoring platforms connect social groups differently (family, friends, call centre workers and social workers)? Like many tables, the most important comparisons and combinations may lie slightly outside what is tabulated in the rows and columns shown. Diagonal contrasts across the table might be more important than any illusion of synoptic completeness, but we want Table 0.1 to illuminate some of the possible contrasts and connections.

Layers of biosensing practice

Across the plural and problematic realities of health, the rows of Table 0.1 locate the cultural, political, economic and institutional layers of biosensing practice. Although in each chapter we deal with specific biosensors as devices – ovulation monitors, falls monitors, cortisol tests and DNA microarrays – we begin here with a preliminary observation: it is impossible to find a biosensor in isolation. Like tools or bodies, they always belong severally to a collective or an assemblage.[1] Biosensors only work when configured within a heterogeneous array of other devices, systems, materials and organisation. A falls monitor, the device that some people (are asked to) wear to detect when they fall over, requires not only a communication infrastructure – a telephone or Internet connection – but usually a telecare monitoring centre that can initiate action in response to a fall should one be detected. Nowadays, there is likely to be an app and a web portal for family and friends, not to mention a call-centre software platform running in the background, logging, scheduling, monitoring and dashboarding its way to efficiency. A fertility monitor, which could be a worn basal body thermometer, might be linked to a mobile phone app, a team of remote experts accessing a database of readings and an analytics interface, and an online discussion

---

[1]   We use 'assemblage' in a loose sense to refer to negotiated mixtures of people and things, artefacts and organisations, stuck together by associating and substituting signs and things (Latour, 1992).

forum. None of these elements, not even the biosensing device itself, is straightforward.

It is not particularly useful, therefore, to regard biosensors as technologies in the sense of the engineering application of science to practical problems. Much of biosensing concerns what happens to the data, how they are understood and how they intersect with or escape other forms of knowledge and expertise. An engineering perspective struggles to accommodate how biosensing might become 'technologies of self' (Rettberg, 2014), techniques of working on self in order to attain certain states of body and mind. In any case, as we will soon argue, biosensors increasingly operate within platform environments in which problems of regulation, property, ethics, inclusion and control are writ large for self and other, for individual and collective, for citizen, customer, corporation and state.

Not only are biosensors woven into a fabric of practice, things and places, but the core biosensing operation of indicating something about the health state of a body cannot always be reliably accomplished. Biosensing faces difficulties rooted deeply in health. Doctors and scientists, among other people, measure physiological states from time to time. Physiological states – temperatures, blood hormone levels connected with stress and levels of DNA expression affecting drug metabolism – are routinely understood as measurable signs of health. However, no exactness, comprehensiveness or sheer volume of physiological data can exhaust the existential inexactness of health. Health can be parameterised in terms of norms – of body temperature, cholesterol levels, cortisol levels, heart rate, blood pressure and so on – that derive from many measurements of observations. However, experience of health or illness, even a life with chronic illness or disability, has no fixed constants, exact parameters or laws. One person's experience of chronic incapacity may well correspond in terms of physiological observations to another's experience of well-being. George Canguilhem's (1989: 201, 199) working definition of health as 'a feeling of assurance in life

7

to which no limit is fixed' and illness or disease as 'a reduction in the margin of tolerance for the environment's inconstancies' implies that experiences of health may diverge from physiological 'constants' or averages derived from accumulated measurements (usually of populations). To take an example that might not be straightforward, cortisol levels do not go up for all people under stress. As we detail in Chapter 2, for some people in distress, cortisol levels go down.

Added to the indeterminacy of health measurement, the lines between body and environment are blurred. Bodies are so plurally entangled in the world that it sometimes hardly makes sense to speak of them as separate from an environment. Concepts of body, skin, self, life, memory, matter, differences, knowledge and action (to list just a few) developed over decades of research in feminist theory, science and technology studies, and cultural anthropology (for example, Barad, 2007; Bennett, 2009) have become radically ecological. We might imagine (see Chapter 4) someone falling out of a chair as a paradigmatic case of a clear and distinct change in body state that could be sensed by a device. It remains, however, a challenge to build a wearable biosensor that can reliably distinguish between someone slowly sitting down and someone sliding off their chair onto the floor. As we write, it seems that the latest Apple Corporation watch, with a biosensor for falls, cannot detect someone jumping off a 17-foot climbing wall (Chen, 2018). The general challenge for biosensing derives from the indeterminacy of the line between body and not-body/environment. Does sliding from a chair to the floor constitute a fall or an intended change in position? It keeps getting worse for biosensing. The act of measuring stress or even a basic physiological variable such as blood pressure changes bodies. Furthermore, the biological integrity of the human body seems to be on the edge of disintegration. We might think of the human microbiome as a remarkably deep-acting internal environment, modulating immune system responses and inflammation reactions, as well as making it possible for us to accomplish elementary feats such as eating.

The indeterminacy of body-environments cascades difficulties for the biosensors. Devices have to be coordinated with each other (hence the many biosensing practices that work by assembling measurements of many bodies). Their results/measurements/indications have to be analysed, interpreted and re-situated amid experiences of health and disease, as well as programmes of action and different forms of expertise and judgement. The devices become products not in their own right, but within arrangements that depend on groups and communities of practice, especially in the form of platforms such as social media. Platforms, institutions, social groups and modes of knowledge are just some of the different facets that unfold around the devices, even if the devices, as triumphs of miniaturisation or intelligence, often seem to be increasingly, sometimes disconcertingly, autonomous.

We have no simple way of conceptualising the diversity of biosensing practices because the lives that they pertain to, actually and potentially, are inherently diverse and indeterminate. This is not to say that biosensors and biosensing practices thwart normalisation. Medical and health institutions and forms of expertise are usually criticised, at least in the humanities and social sciences, for their normalising gaze – for their propensity to observe, measure and classify people ('cases') according to measures of population-level variations. Biosensing often acts normatively; that is, acts to intensify existing norms defined by biopolitical and neoliberal governmentality, with its population measures and controls. One could present a Foucauldian analysis of this tendency running through much contemporary biosensing practice, from fitness to environmental monitoring, in which normalising statements would be webbed into the production of well bodies, active in maintaining their capacity to work and to consume. The vertical axis of Table 0.1

is effectively a gradient of organisational configurations (ranging from localised devices and measurements to institutions and knowledges, from technical operations to statements) that could contribute to the normalisation of vital properties of attributes of citizens, patients, workers and consumers. Fitness, self-health, social care and clinical medicine are not in any relation of degree to each other, although we might say that they range between health (fitness) and disease (social care and clinical medicine), and that biosensing forms part of a discursive formation enunciating subject positions, constituting objects of knowledge and action, and defining gradients of agency and control. Announcements by some life insurers in the US that they would only issue insurance to customers wearing continuously monitored biosensors for heart rate and health are clear statements of intentions to normalise (Baryln, 2018).

Even as they normalise bodies and experiences, biosensing practices that count or record some state of activity such as steps or heart rate can diverge greatly from coordinated programmes of action executed more or less coherently by institutions or large organisations such as health-care providers or hospitals. A platform designed and constructed to gather, aggregate and circulate biosensing data, such as the online ovulation monitoring systems or the social media-enabled DNA genotyping services we discuss in later chapters, differ greatly from the clinical settings in which such biosensing might otherwise take place, creating niches in the broader formations of biomedicalisation, normal and pathological, and disease and health. We will discuss some of the emergences of biosensing in detail in the chapters that follow, but for now, Table 0.1 serves to highlight the very different ecologies of biosensing, and to highlight the need for broad lines of questioning and a re-conceptualisation of biosensors in which frequently used terms such as 'health', 'device', 'bodies' and 'data' are not treated as single or static concepts, but figured as plural and contingent.

Box 0.1: Studying biosensors with Intel Labs

By Celia Roberts, Adrian Mackenzie and Maggie Mort

Throughout this book, we include text boxes about the ethnographic studies underpinning each chapter. Here, we want to insert an almost empty box in recognition of our time spent at Intel with Dawn Nafus and the other researchers, from Intel and from UK and US universities, on the Biosensors in Everyday Life programme. Over four years, we met via teleconference, online and face to face to discuss biosensing and Intel's interest in this area. Some of us visited Intel Labs in California and in Oregon, and two of our students – Joann Wilkinson and Mette Kragh-Furbo – spent a six-week internship in Oregon. All three of us travelled to Intel Labs outside Dublin one freezing week just before Christmas. Hosted by the anthropologist David Prendergast, we discussed biosensing and ageing research, and were thrilled not only to share in a corporate festive meal, but to tour the 'fab' where Intel chips are made.

Our investigation did not involve an ethnographic study of Intel, but we kept wishing it did. It was fascinating to be invited, even briefly, into the corporate hi-tech world and to meet the engineers, scientists, designers and decision-makers, as well as the anthropologists and psychologists working with them. We learnt a lot about our own practices – basically, that we are very slow – and about the multiple and complex ways in which corporations use research in making design and investment decisions. We got a glimpse of the technological iceberg – of the many roads that do not get taken as well as those that start to materialise. There are great stories here, but we cannot tell them.

Biosensors multiply

Our approach to biosensing – somewhat differently to other work that emphasises practices of consumption (Lupton, 2014; Davies, 2015; Harris et al, 2016), surveillance associated with devices and services (Kenner, 2008; Rettberg, 2014), the regulation of medical technologies (Faulkner, 2009), or the politics of health expectations and hopes (Petersen, 2015) – attends to the significance of both the 'bio' and 'sensing' in biosensing practice. 'Bio' has several different resonances in this book. A 'bio' in the sense of a biography, a detailed account of the beginnings, course and ends of a perhaps incomplete life, is definitely part of many of the practices we describe. Every biosensor we discuss – ovulation monitors, falls detectors, cortisol tests, heart-rate monitors and DNA genotyping – inscribes lives within biographies, within stories of major events and intimate experiences, albeit not necessarily in the standard forms of the biographical genre. If we understand health as a set of securities in the present and assurances for the future, then we can expect biographical narratives to be of considerable importance in relation to both experiences of continuity and disruption (Bury, 1982). The life course itself might end up flowing differently, being widened or constricted by tracking and testing. We can imagine a life course being nudged, jolted and marked by its biosensings.

Every biosensor also has a direct relation to 'bio' in the sense of *bios*, the organised form of life on which biomedicine and biopolitical governmentality concentrate in the management of populations of individuals (Foucault, 1990; Rose, 2007). It may be worth considering, we suggest, how biological processes continually exceed or overflow the biological knowledges that are meant to model and structure them as knowable. When we begin to understand biosensors and biosensing as experimental arrangements (especially in their sometimes novel collective formations), we also envisage the possibility that biological concepts change in biosensing practice. Karen Barad's work on the entwining of concept and experiment in quantum physics provides useful theoretical guidance here. As she writes: 'in the absence of appropriate experimental arrangements, concepts do not have determinate meanings' (Barad, 2007: 296). The point here, and one that has often been made in the social studies of science, is that biological concepts, like scientific concepts more generally, depend on experimental apparatus for their grounding. Devoid of experimental or clinical apparatus, concepts lose material relevance. Biosensings may have the capacity to put existing physiological concepts back into an experimental setting via collective arrangements that, as yet, scarcely appear scientific. This may explain the differences between the many scientists actively engaging with biosensing practices and the medical clinicians who approach them warily (West et al, 2017).

Biosensing, we found in some of our cases, prepares the ground for an extension of clinical medicine into everyday life. In projects that seek to aggregate DNA genotyping data and to connect them to other biosensor data (for example, the fitness tracking and genotyping project Infinome [Infinome, 2018]), novel hybridisations of different senses of 'bio' might be in play. Whether in the form of a susceptibility to disease detected by a genetic test (Rose, 2007), or in the promise of a transformed relation to self (as in the quantified self-related sleep, diet and exercise tracking practices described in Neff and Nafus [2016]), biosensors inevitably hybridise different senses of 'bio'.

'Sensing' too has multiple resonances. The term 'sensor' conveys an image of a discrete device, measuring or detecting changes in bodies and environments: steps, falls, heart beats, blood sugar, cortisol concentrations or DNA variants. But the image of a discrete device measuring or observing falls, genetic risks or physiological changes is inadequate to understand sensing practices. Living bodies are full of sensings. What might be called biosensing practices go hand in hand with life in general. Hormones such as cortisol, as we will see in Chapter 2, are themselves biosensors that detect and signal changes in bodily state. To have (or be) a body, to experience in the widest sense of that term, is perhaps a matter of sensing practice, of plural 'heterogeneities doing things' (Bennett, 2009: 122). If bodies sense, then biosensing devices are a provisionally stabilised version of what variously takes place in bodies all the time. The question of whether a biosensor is in us or outside, whether biosensing is something a body does or something done to a body, remains open to reconfiguration. As the philosopher William James (1976: 139) puts it: '"outer" and "inner" are names for two groups into which we sort experiences according to the way in which they act upon their neighbours'. His argument implies that biosensing is already part of what it means to be alive. Biosensing devices are 'outer' sortings of experiences that could just as well be 'inner', or the object of attention of some subject. What happens when biosensing becomes an 'outer' experience? A new observer is arranged. A device to observe bodies, even the ostensibly simple movements of a body taking steps or falling over, presents an experience of observing for someone or something – the observer – for whom the body steps or falls. Biosensors as devices in the strict sense always sense for an observer, even if that observer happens to be the one who bears the biosensor. A basic question for any biosensor follows: for whom does the biosensor sense? As we will see in the chapters that follow, some quite radically different organisations and institutions are shaped around different answers to that question.

If biosensing practices combine the multiple senses of 'bio' and sensing introduced here, we might expect biosensors themselves to be relatively plural and actually difficult to strictly define or delimit. (We refer readers again to Table 0.1 where these different facets of biosensing are laid out.) We might expect biosensing to be complicated by different expectations, to be animated by speculative investments (especially as an outgrowth of 'biocapital', the financial investment in biomedical technologies and techniques such as stem cell therapies and so-called 'biological' drugs from the 1990s onwards [Sunder Rajan, 2006]), to be riven by controversies in the wake of competing claims for significance and veracity (we see this particularly around DNA genotyping biosensing practices), and to be materially diverse in their configurations and implementations. It might be that the forms of knowing they afford and their relation to existing forms of regulation (for instance, of confidentiality or anonymity) will be contentious. In drawing together some diverse instances of biosensing practice in this book, we aim to map the frictions in the 'cultural logic' of biosensing (Nafus, 2013). By exploring how falls, saliva or the temperature of a body wend their way across wearable motion sensors, DNA spotted on a glass plate, a camera lens, the thermocouple of a thermometer or the antibodies on an immunoassay strip (cortisol testing), and then into online platforms with their databases, informational retrieval mechanisms and programmable user interfaces, proliferating across apps and forums and connecting to monitoring centres and sometimes clinics, where distributed forms of action and knowledge come into play, we intend to map this pluralising experience.

These overflows and multiplications are not always immediately visible, and they sometimes develop gradually. For instance, Fitbit users track steps, heart rate and sleep time over extended periods. Some people maintain an active interest in these measurements because they have a weight-loss programme, compete with other people or participate in organised exercise. However, other people lose interest in their steps or their heart rate. Some Fitbit devices continue to sync data with other devices such as tablets and phones, and with the Fitbit platform (see: www.fitbit.com), regardless of wearers' awareness, interest or participation. Fitbit biosensing data pools and aggregates at the platform level, allowing new biosensing observations to take shape. Yahoo Finance recently published an analysis of many billion hours of Fitbit data (Pogue, 2018). The analysis presents patterns of heart-rate variability in different parts of the world, and at different times of the year. Like many conventional studies of heart disease, this data showed variation in heart rates across ethnic groups. Less conventionally, however, it also demonstrated that significant cultural events – Christmas, Easter, Thanksgiving, Divali, Eid al–Fitr, Passover and so on – raise the heart rates of whole populations for several weeks at a time. Whether or not these findings are relevant or important, novel regimes of observation are taking shape through proliferating and distributed biosensing. The cultural-material-lived logic of biosensing cuts across relatively separate domains of telecare, genotyping, cortisol tests and ovulation monitoring in different ways. As the rows of Table 0.1 indicate, the pluralising logics of biosensing practice mean that analytical work will need to consider different layers of practices, as well as the horizontal spectrum of different domains. The 150 billion hours of heart-rate data accrued on the Fitbit platform is only one instance among very many of the data economies surrounding biosensors. The case of the 23andMe genotyping service, which we discuss in Chapter 3, is another, as is the data collected through menstrual-tracking apps such as Clue, discussed in Chapter 1.

The biosensing health platform economies of 'my' and 'our' data

We started from a definition of a biosensor as a device that 'indicates' body or environmental state and biosensing practice as the use of information technology to understand something about indications of body-environment state. Biosensor devices and information technology, particularly in their contemporary instances, are far more extensively enmeshed than these rather flat definitions suggest. The enmeshing often takes the form of a platform, an infrastructurally layered zone where relations between different groups are figured and configured. From a platform perspective, biosensors are just one component in a multilayered assemblage that pulls together web user interfaces, databases, apps, servers, developers, designers, algorithms, engineers, scientists and computer infrastructures, among others. Biosensors generate data, but the act of using, wearing, configuring, observing or monitoring a biosensor is caught in a dense network of relations, many of which might not be immediately visible in the device or adjacent interfaces that have recently tended towards graphically simple, swipey, bright, touch-controlled, animated aesthetics.

Information technology, in the form of mobile devices and their platform support, is used to 'understand' the data, but understanding encompasses a broad range of modalities, many of which unfold across platforms. Sometimes, understanding is mundane and individual. A simple display of heart rate might be all that it entails. In other cases, understanding is highly leveraged through predictive inferences constructed on the basis of models, for instance, as in: the results reported for DNA genotyping, which rely on the statistical models underpinning genome-wide association studies; the falls detectors that now rely on machine-learning algorithms (Pannurat et al, 2014); the 'individualized predictions' of the Clue menstrual-tracking app (Clue, 2018); or the boson-detection models repurposed in the 'Natural Cycles' fertility-tracking app (Scherwitzl et al, 2015). Very often, what felt like personal data is indirectly aggregated and subsumed into other data sets, as Kate Crawford, Jessa Lingel and Tero Karppi (2015) describe in their account of wearable self-tracking devices. Fitabase illustrates one version of a platform mode of understanding: 'Your Participants, Your Data, Your Platform' (Fitabase, 2018). Fitabase aggregates data from many wearable devices and allows researchers to 'stay on top of participant compliance'. The 'self-knowledge' on offer on many of the self-tracking devices is only one side of the platform story. It is very difficult to even approach the topic of biosensors without reference to platform-centred transformations in data practices in science, commerce, industry, government and civil society, as well as without reference to what might be termed the biosensing platform health economy (to conflate just a few different concerns!). Almost every aspect of data, every attribute of it as a conventional, material, epistemic, transactional, administrative or governmental form, undergoes transformation under platform conditions. Some authors call this transformation 'platformisation' (Helmond, 2015; Plantin et al, 2016). Others go so far as to speak, with some justification, of 'platform capitalism' (Srnicek, 2016). In following chapters, we discuss some of the transformations in the context of biosensing.

Given the platform realities of contemporary information technology, the term 'our data' highlights a keystone issue for biosensing. How data becomes – or doesn't become – 'my', 'our', 'their' or 'your data' is a litmus test for a range of localised difficulties, ambivalences, exploits and experiments associated with biosensors and biosensing. Data sharing slips into data owning. The questions of what it means for data to be 'ours' individually or collectively, and what we possess or own of the data, are currently matters of broad social and economic struggle, involving many actors ranging from nation states to data activists, from corporations to patients and citizens. The stakes in these struggles are bound up with platform politics more generally. Structural-level problems concerning regimes of transparency, veracity, property, work and discrimination abound here, as do possibly new practices of care and constitution of self. We need only think of the strange contrasts in sensitivities to health records and social media data – people seem sensitive to any attempts to aggregate and marketise health data, but relatively indifferent to the mundane data-mining of their everyday lives by social media platforms – to recognise that platform data economies have complicated variations and affordances. Although we do not wish to bracket out or sidestep problems of ownership, surveillance, control, neoliberal governmentality or commercial exploitation, we will suggest that biosensing data has some specificities in terms of social groups, institutions, interventions and knowledges that are worth attending to.

In a citizens' panel we conducted in Lancaster, UK, in 2013, discussions took place concerning fertility monitoring and personal genetic tests (Mort et al, 2016; see also Chapters 1 and 3). The most animated of the discussions concerned the problem of 'our' data. The plural possessive 'our' rather than the singular possessive 'my' was notably common. Around the time of the panel, the National Health Service (NHS) in England had launched the 'care.data' campaign (NHS, 2013), a project to aggregate or 'share' all general practice patient records to create a data set capable of supporting data-intensive biomedical research. The campaign went badly wrong when many of the 22 million households in England did not receive the explanatory leaflet and many other people objected to the very idea of 'care.data'. The project was paused in early 2014 and finally abandoned in 2016 after many GPs opted out alongside many patients. In the citizens' panel, 'our' often referred to broad collective groups such as national populations or the group of all patients. In some other settings, as we will see, 'our' might have a more restricted sense relating to groups of people who share a medical condition or a disease, or a group of people related by descent or kinship. In all these settings, 'our' carries a raft of senses of belonging and inclusion.

The term 'our' bears implicit reference to the possibility of dispossession, or data that is 'not ours' because it has somehow become 'theirs'. In biosensing practices, boundaries between 'ours' and 'theirs' are often inscribed by platformising practices that are difficult to negotiate collectively, let alone individually. (Current debates in Europe, North America and Asia concerning the state regulation of social media platforms, as well as the 2018 European Union General Data Protection Regulations, are salient evidence of the difficulty of these fraught negotiations [EU, 2016].) As we will suggest, the constituent subject forms of individuality are being renegotiated in biosensing. The biosensors installed to monitor movements and detect falls in the houses of older people generate data about how those people inhabit their homes, and this sensing informs, for better or worse, plans and actions directly affecting what it means to age, and, indeed, how ageing takes place. Other biosensors and biosensing practices, rather than intensifying the compliance of patients under surveillance to norms, afford deviations and variations from normal treatments or diagnoses (Nafus, 2016b). There are certainly emergent communities of practice around self-tracking, in reanalysis of DNA genotyping data and environmental biosensing practice which suggest that we need not be entirely pessimistic about the outcomes of negotiations around the meaning of data (Sharon, 2018). The ever-present shadowing of 'ours' by its opposite, 'not ours', implies that redefinitions or re-individuations of 'our' will be a particularly important reference point.

The movement of data across platforms suggests that the meaning of 'our data' and its implicit forms of possession, ownership and property have not, and perhaps cannot, stabilise. The regimes of property relations concerned with 'our data' are manifold, complex and power-laden. In England, public opposition to care.data largely concerned risks to the confidentiality of patient–doctor relations, but it also voiced worries about how the integrated data would be used in commercial or industry research and the possible implications for various forms of insurance. Property relations and the forms of ownership associated with data are fraught. As we will see in our exploration of the poorly named 'direct-to-consumer' genetic tests, questions of who owns the data and even whose data is analysed are still very much matters of contestation. As our citizens' panel vocally suggested, being citizens (and data citizens in particular) was just as important as being data consumers or subjects of consumer data. Versions of the problems of platform possession surface not only in our citizens' panel, but also in various ethnographic and media settings. Business models premised on data aggregation vie with cooperative and sometimes socio-political efforts to relocate or migrate data out of the platforms on which it first came into being.

The platform alignments of biosensing

It is not always easy to situate biosensors in relation to bodies and time or, indeed, to life as it is lived individually, in groups or in communities. Data, in the pluralities of its creation, production, accumulation and transformation, is the tissue that potentially connects body states to experiential or experimental understanding, but it connects them ambiguously, loosely and partially. Only exceptionally does the data from a biosensor afford immediate unambiguous observation, understanding or actions in relation to bodies and self. Usually, data has to be collected, accumulated, transformed, rendered in graphical form, subjected to analytical processes of modelling, assimilated to other data sources or interpreted in the light of scientific and clinical knowledges that introduce a welter of assumptions, presuppositions, representations and norms with them. Biosensor data hardly ever aligns directly with experience in any of its modalities. It has to be worked on, and this work is porous, distributed and expansive.

A major concern of this book is to depolarise some of the debates over passive versus active agency in understanding biosensor data. How do we hold in focus the agencies that range from the mildly active consumption of wearable gadgets and apps to highly activated collectives or communities of biosensing? We address this problem by attending to the platform configurations of biosensing practice. Platforms are the main place where agency problems play out, and where the expansive, distributed and connective work of understanding can take place. Collectives sometimes emerge on the edges of or between platforms. However, we lack good understandings of platform biosensing.

In better understanding the platform realities of biosensing, the concept of biomedical platform proposed by Paul Keating and Alberto Cambrosio (2003), in *Biomedical platforms: Realigning the normal and the pathological in late-twentieth-century medicine*, offers an important lead. Scientific and clinical knowledges, practices and value regimes do not and cannot coincide precisely because health – in any of the guises typified in the columns of Table 0.1 – is a 'feeling of assurance' (Canguilhem, 1989: 201), not a norm prescribed by biological processes. (For biology, a disease is biologically just as normal as the absence of illness.) Keating and Cambrosio, departing from Canguilhem's (1989) philosophical account of the non-alignment between biology and medicine and between the normal and the pathological, define biomedical platforms as 'material and discursive arrangements that act as the bench upon which conventions concerning the biological or normal are connected with conventions concerning the medical or the pathological' (Keating and Cambrosio, 2003: 332).

Keating and Cambrosio suggest that biomedical platforms, especially the quasi-automated imaging and testing instruments now common in hospital pathology labs and clinics, take shape at the intersection of different knowledge practices coming out of biology and medicine. Biomedical platforms for assaying or imaging tissue samples are not scientific or clinical instruments like a thermometers or scales. Although they certainly incorporate measurements and observations, biomedical platforms do more than measure or observe. (Through an extended case study of how cell flow cytometry machines moved to the centre of HIV/AIDs diagnosis and monitoring, Keating and Cambrosio illustrate differences between scientific instruments and biomedical platforms.) They extend beyond measurement or observations 'insofar as they embody regulations and conventions of equivalence, exchange and circulation' (Keating and Cambrosio, 2003: 324). Biomedical platforms encompass regulations, standards or conventions concerning what counts as a clinically valid measurement, or apply categories and clusterings derived from clinical experience in their technical operations (algorithms, classifications or implementations of rules in code). The 'material and discursive arrangements' or 'configurations' (Suchman, 2012) of platforms align the different realities of biological and medical knowledge practices. They locally stabilise the zone of slippage that runs between biological accounts of living things and medical accounts of disease or illness as pathology. They establish rapprochements between experimental configurations concerned with forms of life and regulated clinical expertise concretised around norms of disease and illness.

Biomedical platforms that image, test, diagnose or monitor illness rely on prior negotiations and alignments of different knowledge practices. (Current efforts to establish precision medicine based largely on genomic science and its sequencing platforms are another example.) Although biology and medicine thereby connect in many respects (as highlighted in the accounts of biomedicalisation presented by Adele Clarke et al [2010]), we will propose that the irreducibility of illness, disease and health experience to biology is also vital to biosensing.[2] The negotiation of different approaches to living (and living data) coming from biology and medicine underpins wide-ranging cultural logics of biosensing.

Biosensors and biosensing have a complex relation to pre-existing biomedical platforms such as medical scanners. The non-coincidence between biology and medicine affects biosensing in manifold ways. Although biosensing is not regulated by the conventions and standards applicable to biomedical platforms, its platforms also cross over between biology and health. In order to respect the specificities of both the life sciences and medicine, and to register the importance of various practices and technologies that bridge between them, we pay close attention in this book to platform alignments, forms of regulation and convention associated with biosensors, and configurations that assemble or address different biological and clinical knowledges. In our different case studies – stress, fertility monitoring, telecare and personal genetic testing – we explore the ramifications of the

---

[2]   In our observations, the idea of biomedicine, which legitimates the institutional and industrial convergence of medicine and biology, tends to cover over the emergent realignments of science and medicine. Clarke et al's (2010) more sociological thesis of biomedicalisation at least points to some of the practices of alignment, but it tends to elide the constitutive differences of biology and medicine in order to highlight the informatics and industrial elements of contemporary medicine.

biology–medicine fault line as it runs through the handling and management of data, the different social groupings, expertises and networks taking shape, and the struggles over what counts as knowledge and for whom.

Norms are a sticky issue for biosensing platforms. Illness is often clinically evaluated through norms or statistical measures of central tendencies in populations. These norms are embedded in biomedical platforms as part and parcel of their diagnostic operation. Such norms have a much more tenuous presence on biosensing platforms. The obvious example in our group of case studies would be the genetic tests. They often rely on non-clinical genomic research (especially genome-wide association studies, as discussed in Chapter 4), whose clinical significance (and statistical significance) cannot be easily mapped onto individual experiences of illness or health. The fact that the significance of biosensor data, even in the vast quantities produced by contemporary DNA genotyping devices, cannot be immediately evaluated in terms of health and disease triggers more complex attempts to probe around, to find signals or patterns within the data that could, even if only in the future, be clinically significant. Personalised medicine is one such organisational attempt to render biology more clinically relevant (Tutton, 2016). In extreme cases, and for some of the biosensing we discuss, avalanches of data flow untapped, un-enacted, un-understood in big data un-analytics.

What does tracking the internal fault line running through biosensing platforms mean in practice? Sometimes, biosensing attempts to test connections between seemingly unrelated life or health events. From a platform perspective, it is particularly important to attend to the regulatory practices and conventions developing in and around biosensing as it connects different biosensors and aggregates data sets. As we will suggest, these regulatory practices often entail reconfigured relations between individuals and groups, altered arrangements for the circulation of data (data being uploaded, shared and variously distributed as part of its analysis and interpretation), and substantively novel material arrangements for the organisation of practices of monitoring and intervention. Data ownership and property rights are an increasingly important zone of regulatory attention. However, it is not always certain in what regulatory zone biosensing occurs. Sometimes, biosensing practices entrain individuals in a pre-clinical departure zone, queued for imminent proximity with clinical expertise (for instance, ovulation monitoring prepares the ground in various ways for assisted reproductive technologies such as in vitro fertilisation [IVF], and the 'kitemarking' of health-tracking apps by the UK NHS sets up a pre-clinical path [Pym, 2014]). At other times, a medically approved biosensor finds unexpected biosensing uses (an ovulation device approved for contraception might find uses in conception). In any case, the regulatory conventions for many biosensors are not set or fixed in the same way as they might be for accepted clinical medicine and biomedical platforms. For instance, DNA genotyping, despite the intensive involvement of biomedical researchers, still produces highly variable test results, with alarming consequences for participants: one testing service might predict early onset Alzheimer's disease and another might not (Hercher, 2018). In regulatory terms, they function as quasi-biomedical platforms. More dramatically, a biosensing platform might reshape the regulatory regime of existing biomedical platforms: DNA ancestry testing might effectively deregulate existing forms of biomedical governance; and it is possible to use DNA genotyping platforms to sidestep, for instance, the UK regulations pertaining to anonymity protecting egg and sperm donation for use in IVF (Weaver, 2018).

Cultural logics of biosensing

The fact that clinicians often regard biosensor-derived data with suspicion, and biosensing itself as a possible symptom of mental illness or 'begging for diagnosis' (West et al, 2017: 8), is significant. It suggests that biosensing is not at home in the theatres of biomedical practice. The regulatory dynamics at the heart of the platforms animate what Dawn Nafus (2013: xviii) (echoing the work of cultural critic Frederic Jameson [1991] on the 'cultural logic' of late capitalism) calls a 'cultural logic of biosensing'. This logic, Nafus argues, describes how the invention and innovation of biosensors overflows the marketing and product development focused on devices. The fact that most people lose interest in wearable devices after a few days/ weeks/months does not dampen ongoing excitement about their potential to revolutionise individual and public health. From a commercial perspective, the rapid loss of interest is a problem. Viewed from the perspective of a cultural logic of biosensing, gadgets are only part of broader transverse relations that bring disparate people and groups into contact, and platforms might be able to arrange connections that go well beyond the limits of devices as products with defined features.

The cultural logic of biosensing, configured on platforms, operates in the zone of slippage between biological forms in all their rich sensing entanglements and life lived according to norms of intrinsic variability. Biosensing as a platform practice, we somewhat tentatively suggest, culturally realigns biology and medicine around health. We recognise that biomedical research strives to overcome the existential indeterminacies of health and disease experiences by bringing, among other things, biology to bear on disease. We know that medical imaging, clinical trials, stratified medicine, personalised medicine, precision medicine and, in some respects, evidence-based medicine all respond to the inexactness or variability of health – and medical expertise – by treating patients as members of populations. We know too that health is not a measurable object, but a regulatory feeling of the possibilities of reaction to the inconsistencies of environments. It follows that no biosensor, regardless of its precision or accuracy, and regardless of its biological or technical sophistication (including the 'smarts' of machine learning), can by itself make up for the inevitable misalignments between biological laws expressed as statistics (means, ranges, deviations, other measures of population variability and so on) and experiences of health and disease in which any variation can be normative. Biosensing work as understanding will require the comparisons and recalibrations that make sense of the variations in terms of norms. One might think of fitness training or the many tracking practices associated with the Quantified Self movement as occurring in the space of health understood as a feeling of assurance in life. We should add too that it is hard to imagine how biosensing could even up disparities such as the different life expectancies between rich and poor areas.

The implication of the platform realignment argument is not that biosensors are destined to fail as innovations. Gadgets and devices may fall out of fashion, and there may even be large-scale abandonments of certain biosensing trajectories. Rather, the point here is different: biosensing practices, insofar as they concern health broadly construed as the 'regulatory flywheel of possibilities of reaction' (Canguilhem, 1989) or the capacity to bounce back, will be both normative and unstable. They inhabit the uneven terrain where biology and medicine, laboratory and clinic, encounter each other along the meandering fault line of biological processes and medical normalisation, with its classificatory operations. Even as biology strives and sometimes succeeds in measuring states of particular bodies in their subtly varying relations to experimentally accessible environments, medicine grapples with the problem of how to classify varying cases. If clinics, hospitals, pharmaceuticals and medical devices are some of the historically constituted architectures and artefacts of normalising efforts, the wearable devices, apps, research projects and publications crowding around platforms are the emerging architectures and configurations of the biosensing formation.

Summary of the argument: sensing, biology–medicine and platforms

This introduction has climbed through steep terrain. Biosensors and biosensing are problematic on epistemic, economic, institutional and cultural grounds. In this book, we concentrate on bodies experienced in health and disease, ongoing tensions between biological, medical and other body knowledges, and the emerging platforms that reconfigure what it means to 'have' the data. The three themes shaping our account of biosensing can be summarised in terms of:

- the indeterminacies of situated, living, environed bodies sensing and being sensed;
- the slippages of biology and medicine, of science laboratories and medical clinics, as they regulate the incommensurabilities of life as biological form and life as lived experience; and
- the gathering of data by devices and on platforms that align and configure experiences of health.

Overview of chapters

The case studies we explore in the chapters could be seen to follow the lifespan, from ovulation monitoring, to childhood and adult stress, through practices of prediction viewing genetic risk, to systems of remote or automated care for frail older people. We could have chosen many other case studies, such as home foetal heart monitoring or home dopplers, infectious disease biosensors, diabetes management, or military personnel monitoring. We chose case studies spanning significant experiences, events and durations throughout life. Some punctuate and others mark epochs of a life. Ultimately, they concern the lineaments of a life course.

Chapter 1 explores contemporary uses of fertility and sex hormone biosensing, asking how their use is rearticulating sex/gender, sexuality and reproduction. Working with findings from Joann Wilkinson's ethnography of ovulation monitoring and our citizens' panel, and with textual materials about these kinds of biosensing, we critically analyse emerging practices around reproduction and sex/gender, asking how the collection and analysis of personal data is entangled with corporate biodigital platforms, and with feminist and other forms of collective politics.

Stress biosensing is the focus of Chapter 2. Beset by the notable complexities of titrating or measuring stress (either via so-called 'stress hormones', by heart rate or by galvanic skin response), these practices remain rather undeveloped compared to fertility biosensing. However, due to pre-existing narratives about stress and mental health and function (for example, found in literatures on childhood trauma and workplace stress), information about an individual's stress and the collation of such information about particular groups is potentially of interest to many groups, including employers, foster carers and social services, and the military. We argue here that information about biological changes thought to be related to stress is only valuable if triangulated with other information about the person's situation, including psychosocial histories and historical and geographical location.

Analysing data from our citizens' panel work in Chapter 3, we explore how citizens make sense of such information, and whether, when and how knowing about future health risk might be desirable. How do citizens and users make sense of the complexities of genomic science that such devices bring them into contact with? How does direct-to-consumer genetic testing alter our perceptions of health, reproduction, families and futurity? DNA genotyping is a form of biosensing concerned with genetic risks, susceptibilities and relatedness. This chapter argues that genotyping services such as 23andMe prompt us to take seriously the platform realities of biosensing. DNA genotyping platforms attempt to aggregate data on an unprecedented scale, to anchor the significance of DNA variations for health and kinship, and to connect DNA variations to health practices and health futures. The biosensors commonly used in DNA genotyping are microarrays. The amount of data that they produce poses challenges for biosensing. The Internet platforms and products associated with direct-to-consumer DNA genotyping embody a personalising approach to health and medicine, even though the connections between underpinning scientific findings concerning genomic variation and clinical interventions or treatments are mostly tenuous. At the same time, because the significance of the million or so variations reported in a typical DNA genotype is mostly undefined, the data has led to many individual and collective attempts to create new connections, to experiment with novel collective forms of analysis and treatment, and to build new relations between biology, medicine and everyday life.

How does biosensing reach into the lives of older people living at home? In Chapter 4, we examine care monitoring systems for older people, or 'telecare', as this has become known. We focus on the wearable falls detector – an alarm device that triggers, it is claimed, when a person trips or falls. We explore findings from ethnographies of home telecare and from citizens' panel debates on how individuals and families live with such systems, and how falls detectors are constructed as workable. Following individuals' interactions with telecare, we question the notion of self-tracking in this context, preferring the term 'dys-tracking' as better reflecting their relationship with automated devices. Falls detectors are technically highly complex, collecting data that is difficult to interpret. Ageing bodies are invariably assessed as low functioning and intrinsically at risk. Views from our citizens' panels, however, show a more active and imaginative constituency, where practices of self-care exist alongside or in parallel with remote-care systems.

The Conclusion focuses on the gap between two prominent public narratives of health biosensing: the promissory-horizon narratives that biosensing will soon solve many important and intractable problems; and the disappointment, overhype narrative, which suggests that biosensing often fails to deliver on its promise, and that users give up on their devices or use them only for narcissistic ends. We argue that research, policy and practice (everything from technology design to clinical medicine and health-related activism) would do well to pay attention to the 'bio' in all its senses and to platforms, recognising all the ways that we are living data and that data is lively.

1

Fertility Biosensing

Bodies constantly sense and humans frequently notice their bodies in order to promote or protect health. Lying at the heart of human life, reproduction has long been entwined with both kinds of sensing. Contemporary fertility biosensing blends techniques of body awareness and related forms of recording (such as diaries and charts) with modern forms of scientific and biomedical knowledge, high-tech gadgets and biodigital platforms. Recent studies show that people who menstruate and/or have ovaries and a uterus[1] use a wide variety of technologies – from paper-based diaries, through mobile phone apps, to wearable biosensing devices – to track and record fertility or sex hormone-related events such as menstruation, ovulation, unprotected heterosexual intercourse and other acts of insemination (Lupton, 2015; Wilkinson et al, 2015; Epstein et al, 2017).

Fertility biosensors articulate bodies that menstruate and/or ovulate through codifications of cycles, relying on an organisation of time across days, notably, the notion of a regular 28-day cycle and 'peak fertile times'. Fertility biosensors are only relevant for

---

[1]   It is important to note that people who do not identify as women or girls can have ovaries and uteruses, and may menstruate, and equally to acknowledge that not everyone who identifies and/or lives as a woman or girl has a uterus, ovaries or female genitalia, or, indeed, may menstruate or ovulate. Language is struggling to catch up with these increasingly public facts. In this chapter, we attempt to be non-discriminatory and specific in our choice of words and to highlight and explore the ways in which biosensing discourses, devices and practices both facilitate and inhibit the expansion and proliferation of sex and gender in contemporary cultures.

a certain portion of one's life: the so-called 'reproductive years' (which can, of course, constitute many decades). Menstrual apps marketed to young women and those oriented towards tracking the (peri-)menopause help to constitute the beginnings and ends of this period of time, as well as shaping its contemporary unfolding as a biomedical phenomenon. In this sense, they directly participate in the figuring (that is, both the discursive formation and the lived experience) of women's (and potentially men's and others') life courses more broadly. As the so-called new reproductive technologies did before them (Franklin, 2013), fertility biosensors, in other words, remake what it means to be sexed/gendered, to reproduce and, thus, to be human.

Reasons for monitoring fertility and associated flows of sex hormones are diverse, ranging from curiosity, through strong desires to avoid or achieve pregnancy, to medical concerns about gynaecological or reproductive health (endometriosis, polycystic ovary syndrome and other conditions), and the tracking of processes of gender transition. In this chapter, we explore practices of fertility and sex hormone biosensing, asking how they are changing enactments of contemporary bodies, sex/gender, reproductive relations and associated notions of 'the reproductive years'.

Fertility tracking also increasingly takes place on digital platforms amid wider cultural logics of biosensing. While most fertility-tracking apps and devices are marketed as consumer goods and services, they also have contested multiple links to biomedicine and clinical spaces. In 2017, for example, Swedish start-up Natural Cycle managed to get their fertility-tracking app registered in the US and Europe as a medical device after clinical trials demonstrated its effectiveness as a contraceptive (Natural Cycles, 2018).[2] In this chapter, then, we also examine

---

[2] For analysis of the ways in which health biosensing has challenged conventional biomedical device and data regulation in the US, see Fiore-Gartland and Neff (2016).

how data from fertility monitoring is collected, analysed and debated within biodigital health platform economies and how links between fertility- and sex hormone-related biosensing and biomedicine are imagined and enacted.

As mentioned in the Preface, our initial response to Intel Labs proposed three linked projects: an ethnographic study of direct-to-consumer genetic testing; an ethnographic study of fertility monitoring; and a citizens' panel to deliberate on the findings of these studies and to consider biosensing in society more broadly. At the time, there was only sparse social-scientific work on fertility monitoring and very little discussion of it in public forums. There was, however, a substantial social-scientific and feminist literature on in vitro fertilisation (IVF), ovulation and (in)fertility, to which one of us (Celia Roberts) had contributed for some years (Roberts and Franklin, 2004; Franklin and Roberts, 2006; Throsby and Roberts, 2010). The project on fertility monitoring, then, was framed to develop this critical feminist trajectory in recognition of the ever-increasing significance of (in)fertility as a global health and social issue. Joann Wilkinson's ethnographic study, as summarised in Box 1.1, explored ovulation biosensing as a contemporary practice that bridges the sometimes highly fraught (and culturally very densely symbolised) temporal gap between the formation of an intention to become pregnant and actually conceiving. Focusing on heterosexual cis-women[3] wishing to have a child, Wilkinson studied the use of biosensing devices by women who had not experienced fertility problems and those who had, employing face-to-face interviewing, online ethnographic methods (analysing women's participation in online fertility forums) and textual analysis of related materials such as biosensor manufacturers' websites and promotional videos and leaflets as her key research methods (Wilkinson et al, 2015; Wilkinson,

---

[3]   'Cis-women' refers to people who have been figured medically and socially as female since birth and who self-identify as women as adults.

2016). Here, we explore the rapid expansion of fertility monitoring (and associated social-scientific analysis) that has occurred since 2014, situating Wilkinson's ethnographic findings in the wider contemporary context of other fertility- and sex hormone-related biosensing practices. Our assessment of these shifts stems from analysis of accounts of fertility monitoring, including those found in product websites, YouTube vlogs and videos, online discussions, articles in the popular and medical press, and academic literatures. This range allows us to explore the cultural logics of fertility biosensing in their multiplicity and their shared framings.

'Femtech' and the new fertility

Since the inception of IVF in late 1970s' Britain, and its spiralling growth in the 1990s and 2000s as it was rolled out as part of National Health Service (NHS) provision (as well as becoming privately available in many parts of the world), 'fertility' has both developed as a technical object and steadily entered public discourse and the everyday lives of people of reproductive age. Biosensing devices such as worn ovulation monitors, hormone-measuring devices and pregnancy testing kits are an increasingly important part of this emerging (re-)formation of fertility. Both symptom and contributing factor, such devices are, we will argue, deeply entangled in the folded enactments of contemporary reproductive bodies and relations.

As detailed later, in the 1980s, domestic or non-medical fertility tracking was typically either a relatively esoteric self-knowledge practice engaged in by feminists, or part of the 'rhythm' or 'Billings' methods widely promoted by the Roman Catholic Church as morally acceptable forms of contraception. Today, in contrast, while fertility is figured as highly complex, biomedicalised and a site of intervention, it is also something everyday and domestic. Good citizens are expected to know and understand ovulation and menstruation – this is now part of the secondary school science curriculum in England for example – and those who ovulate are expected to actively manage the reproductive and medical implications of this process. While, in many ways, remaining a taboo topic socially, menstruation is also becoming more widely acknowledged and discussed in many parts of the world. This is evident not only in the proliferation of period-tracking apps and online advertising and discussion of new 'hygiene' products (such as 'period-proof' underwear), but also in emerging forms of menstrual activism (Radnor, 2017). Of course, huge disparities still exist with regard to access to information, medical assistance and practical means of managing menstruation, as well as the effects of cultural taboos on daily life. While millions of people are tracking their periods online, many others cannot access basic sanitary products, toilets or running water.

In this chapter, we use the term 'fertility' to refer to a wide range of biopsychosocial processes.[4] 'Fertility and sex-hormone biosensors', then, include devices to monitor or test for ovulation, to measure sperm count, to track menstruation, to test for pregnancy, to trace hormonal changes before, during and after menopause, and even to monitor foetal development. Devices and apps designed for domestic use to address all these aims are currently available in the UK, the US and many other countries. Figure 1.1 maps the range of such devices in 2017, providing brand names and naming the overall group 'femtech'. This figure by no means covers the full range of such devices: a recent survey conducted by Epstein et al shows that there are over 1,000 free smartphone apps to track menstrual patterns (Moglia et al, 2016; Epstein et al, 2017). (Most of these, the authors argue, are scientifically invalid and therefore useless!)

---

[4]   We do not discuss biosensing devices or self-tracking apps designed to address sexual practices unrelated to reproduction (for a discussion of these, see Lupton, 2014).

Figure 1.1: Mapping the 'femtech' market in 2017

Women's Health Market Map

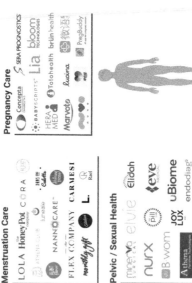

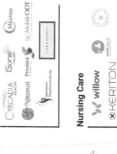

Source: Copyright of CB Insights (www.cbinsights.com/research/report/womens-health-technology-transforming/) (2017)

That most of these apps are free is significant – the owners of smartphones can use them without additional costs. Biosensing devices, however, as described in Box 1.1, come with a variety of price tags and may remain prohibitively expensive for many.

Menstrual tracking is widespread among a range of people, including trans men, gender-queer/fluid and agender individuals, and many groups of women. Ovulation tracking is becoming increasingly popular among those wishing to become pregnant, while semen analysis is also starting to occur outside of conventional medical arrangements (Fox, 2017). While medical research suggests that fertility-tracking apps are 'generally inaccurate' (Setton et al, 2016), their popularity is undeniable, with an estimated 200 million users in 2018 according to journalist Jane Dreaper (2016). Indeed, in the health and fitness arena, they are said to come second only to running apps. These numbers are now raising concerns about people using fertility tracking instead of hormonal or barrier contraceptives (Brigham, 2018; Chaudhuri, 2018; Dreaper, 2016). As Dana Greenfield (2016) notes in her analysis of the Quantified Self movement, many users configure their biosensing as a rejection of biomedical accounts of physical processes and related clinical interventions. Anecdotally, we have learned of people using menstrual tracking to avoid hormonal contraception for health and political reasons, despite medical and public concerns about risks of unwanted pregnancies and/or sexually transmitted infections. The high number of people engaging in fertility monitoring, we suggest, show the ways in which cultural logics of biosensing (specifically, the idea that knowing about one's bodily processes is beneficial for health and well-being) sometimes run against the grain of biomedical knowledge and expertise.

These devices and apps are part of multiple, complex practices and various biomedical and social media platforms. (It is important to note that many apps are not technically biosensors, relying on manual data entry by users rather than directly measuring any bodily flows; however, biosensing platforms typically now include mobile phone apps).[5] Some biosensors, such as sperm-count devices, require users to send biological samples off to laboratories for professional analysis. Others, such as pregnancy-testing kits, are designed for singular or one-off (if sometimes frequent) use at home. Still others, such as the ovulation monitors studied by Wilkinson, are designed to be used regularly while the user is attempting to become (or to avoid becoming) pregnant. Some ovulation devices measure basal body temperature, making the assumption that temperature rises and falls in predictable correlation with ovulation. Others measure hormonal flows, tracking the rise and fall of luteinising hormone (LH) or oestrogen across the ovulation and menstrual cycle. Importantly, as much work in science and technology studies argues (Akrich, 1992; Oudshoorn, 2003), devices can also be used to do something other than that built-in by designers: peri-menopausal people, for example, might use an ovulation biosensor to check their changing hormone levels, as might trans or gender-queer/fluid people wanting to track or experiment with hormonal medications.

Box 1.1: Ovulation biosensing for conception

By Joann Wilkinson

Ovulation biosensors are devices worn on, or used with, the body that can help users detect ovulation. Ranging in price from a few to several hundred pounds sterling, they can be used to measure and detect changing hormone levels either through saliva, urine or temperature. Each of these sensors relies on an

---

[5] The 'Temperature Egg' studied by Wilkinson, for example, originally involved a worn thermometer, a handheld device and a computer interface to remote 'fertility experts'. Since that study was completed in 2015, the company has replaced the handheld device and computer interface with a mobile phone app.

understanding of human reproduction that suggests that a 'surge' of LH and an increase in oestrogen occurs around the time of ovulation.

Within the Billings method, ovulation patterns were assessed through individual measurement or observation and recording of physical signs: changes in vaginal or cervical fluid and basal body temperature (and sometimes also sexual desire). Monitoring basal body temperature requires users to use a thermometer immediately on waking throughout the whole menstrual cycle, and to record this on a monitoring chart. This method is based on the understanding that body temperature is lower in the first half of the cycle than the second. Ovulation takes place at the point of change, observed through a 'dip and sharp rise' on the chart. This method is used retrospectively in order to learn if ovulation has taken place and to gain insight into general ovulatory patterns; it does not predict when ovulation will take place. Contemporary biosensing devices build on this pattern of work, trying to automate the temperature taking and recording through worn thermometers and associated information technology (IT). Importantly, they also use algorithms to predict when ovulation will occur, and provide users with information in advance, so that they can plan their sexual encounters accordingly.

Other fertility biosensing systems directly measure hormones in urine or saliva. One of the most widely used devices includes ovulation testing strips (known in online forums as ovulation predictor kits (OPKs), or 'cheapies' because of their low cost). These flimsy 5–7.5 cm-long strips of card are dipped in urine for approximately 15 seconds to detect the LH surge around the time of ovulation. Positive results (high levels of LH) result in a line as dark as the control line, indicating that ovulation will take place within the following 24–36 hours. More expensive models, such as those offered by Clearblue, encase the strips in plastic and use smiley faces to indicate a positive result.

The 'ovulation microscope' is less commonly used than basal body temperature monitoring or OPKs. Resembling a tube of lipstick, it can be used to detect changing levels of oestrogen in saliva leading up to ovulation. The user places a small amount of saliva on the lens, waits for it to dry and then looks through the microscope, bringing the view into focus as needed. If oestrogen is present in saliva in sufficient quantities, then crystallised ferning patterns will appear on the lens, thus indicating that ovulation is near. This reusable device can be bought online or at a pharmacy for less than £15.

My research was based on interviews with 27 women, five general practitioners and three professionals working in an ovulation biosensor manufacturing company, as well as an online ethnography of reproduction-related forums. I explored how manufacturers of ovulation biosensors tried to align their products with cis-women's practices of trying to conceive, and what happened when these heterosexual cis-women engaged with such devices. I found that manufacturers' claims often related to time. They indicated that women could gain a specific number of 'fertile days', enabling them to plan and prepare time for reproductive heterosex with male partners. Manufacturers also claimed that ovulation biosensors enabled women to take a more targeted approach and thus make up for lost time when trying to conceive 'late' in life. Furthermore, knowing ovulation was presented in these discourses as a single step: a linear process of testing and obtaining clear results.

In contrast, the women in my study found ovulation to be uncertain and frequently changing. Indeed, knowing ovulation was not a single step of testing and obtaining a result, as presented by the manufacturers of biosensor devices. Ovulation data was not 'out there' waiting to be accessed. Instead, knowing ovulation was done through practices: testing and retesting, comparing samples, making conclusions, and collaboratively coding data with other women on online fertility forums. The following post is an example of this:

> This morning I got my 4th flashing smiley face – I really thought that it would be solid by now. I don't really understand how it is supposed to detect hormonal changes each month – when you buy a new pack you get a new holder so it can't be that the tests are getting used to me as a new holder will be like using them for the first time all over again. Also, are you meant to dtd [do the deed] every day while its flashing, and eventually solid? My poor OH [other half] is worn out. It sounds silly but I'm worried he will run dry!! These tests are all new to me, any advice would be much appreciated, thank you. (Post by Fruitcake, Fertility Forum, consulted 7 October 2013: 17:02)

Knowing ovulation meant engaging in scientific practices at home and online. For some women, biosensing was exciting and interesting; they learned new things about their bodies, at least for a period of time:

> I got a high today, got so excited when I saw it [a symbol on the monitor that denotes 'peak fertility' or the day of ovulation]!... Anyone would think I've just found I'm pregnant! Ha! One step closer I guess x. (Post by Minnien, Fertility Forum, consulted 20 November 2013: 14:2)

Knowing ovulation could, however, also generate confusion and even anxiety. Additionally, the multiple tasks that women engaged in as part of biosensing were often invisible to male partners, supporting normative figurations of reproductive heterosexual romance as 'natural' and (ideally at least) 'spontaneous'. The following post highlights these tensions:

> It's hard to be doing it like rabbits when you have stressful jobs.... We were more 2–3 times a month kind so no way we can just forget we are ttc [trying to conceive]. Or I will never get pregnant. My strategy is to chart and use opks etc to reduce the number of times needed to a minimum 😊. (Post by ButterScott, Fertility Forum, consulted 16 August 2013, 11:02)

Practices of ovulation biosensing reconfigure what it means to try to conceive by introducing new stages in the process of trying to do so. These practices then provided women with a framework, either to try out different options, or to move onto the next stage if things did not go to plan. Whereas women's initial practices of trying to conceive were located within an unmarked period of time, engaging with biosensing technologies meant that they came to be defined by new materialities of conception such as 'fertile days', 'LH surge' or ferning patterns on a microscope. These made ovulation more tangible and aligned to particular understandings of time and timing. Women drew on these to create 'conceptive trails', paths along which they tried make sense of ovulation, to calculate their chances of conceiving and to develop theories around why they had not conceived. In interviews and online, women thus articulated the multiple ways in which biosensing was implicated in new responsibilities, labours and anxieties around sexual reproduction.

Citizens talking ovulation

In 2013, we conducted a citizens' panel on biosensing entitled 'Our Bodies, Our Data'. Part of this experiment involved discussion of the 'Temperature Egg' and the 'ovulation microscope', two devices that Wilkinson's research had highlighted as widely used by the women in her sample (the other topic was direct-to-consumer genetic testing, as discussed in Chapter 3). Using Wilkinson's ethnographic findings, we constructed a scenario about a couple who wanted to become pregnant. This scenario is a story based around a family with multiple health-related concerns. Some of the family members turn to different kinds of biosensor for help with these problems. We gave this scenario to the citizen participants at the start of the day.[6] In this, 36-year-old Louise is trying to have a child with her 30-year-old partner, Yusef. They had been trying for a year when Louise decided to purchase an ovulation microscope (£12.99 at the local pharmacy) to learn to track her ovulation. Louise finds using the microscope easy and even exciting, and learns a lot about her ovulatory cycle. She does not become pregnant, however, and so turns to the Internet to research and discuss her situation with other women. Louise reads on the forum about another device called the 'Temperature Egg', a more complex, and expensive, ovulation-tracking device comprised of a body-worn temperature sensor, a handheld device and computer application, and remote access to a set of 'fertility experts' ready and willing to interpret monitoring data and make recommendations about the optimal timing of sexual intercourse. (In our current analysis, the Temperature Egg exemplifies platformised biosensing; the device is an element in a coordinated assemblage of people, databases, expertise and communication and social networks.) In order to facilitate the discussion, we intentionally left the scenario open at that point so that panel members could discuss what might happen if Louise went down that track.

A key element of the citizens' panel method is to invite expert witnesses to be questioned by panel members. In the approach we adopted, these experts were not given the floor to present talks or to set the agenda, but instead asked to answer questions prepared by the panel during the discussion of the scenario, facilitated by us. We invited two experts to perform this role for the fertility scenario: a local General Practitioner (GP) with a special interest in (in)fertility; and the Chief Executive

---

[6]   The full scenario can be found in the Appendix and in the report by the Living Data Research Group (2013).

of Infertility Network UK, a national charity dedicated to the support of people affected by infertility. As we have detailed elsewhere (Living Data Research Group, 2013; Mort et al, 2016), panel members drew on their discussions to formulate a set of questions to these experts about fertility biosensing:

- Are these fertility products regulated in the UK?
- Can you tell that you are ovulating from saliva? Aren't there better ways? Would you agree that 20,000 readings [of temperature, in relation to ovulation] creates an illusion of accuracy?
- Is there a need for better education about fertility?
- How do we know whether we can trust these companies? Is there a trusted website to make sense of other sites?

The panel's discussion and questions, and the ensuing conversation with the experts, indicated a high level of scepticism about the need for technical ovulation monitoring of the sort Wilkinson studied. Panel members were concerned that devices such as the Temperature Egg were unregulated and could be providing users with inaccurate (and therefore unhelpful) results. Indeed, the GP stated that the NHS guidelines do not normally recommend using temperature measurements to assess ovulation stage, despite their long history as part of the rhythm method contraceptive technique. She told the panel that she was unconvinced that 20,000 measurements per day were in any way necessary or helpful for coming to know whether a user was ovulating. The panel discussed lay knowledge of ovulation and whether or not those trying to get pregnant understand the processes of ovulation very well. Although people may have been taught about ovulation at school, the general orientation of sex education is towards avoiding conception. The Chief Executive of Infertility Network UK emphasised the significant role of charities in providing public education about (in)fertility and 'reliable' information about fertility science and related clinical procedures, but also noted the significant funding shortages affecting their activities.

During this debate, the GP declared that she was highly sceptical about the value of ovulation biosensing devices in primary care. She felt that it was unlikely that doctors would be able or willing to use the information gathered through their use, and that clinicians would always insist on standard, one-off tests of ovulation before referring anyone to fertility services. The panel also raised concerns about the decreased funding of public health care, reaffirming the value of free-at-the-point-of-access services. Panel members were concerned that equity of access should be maintained, even if biosensors do become a routine part of care.

The sense that fertility monitoring is out of synch with its clinical relevance is echoed in published literature. In the *American Journal of Maternal/Child Nursing*, for example, Patricia McCartney (2016) writes that although fertility-monitoring apps produce information potentially of interest to nurses working not only on fertility issues, but also on painful or irregular menstruation and various forms of ovulatory diseases, US nurses do not incorporate this information into their clinical questioning. This reluctance is part of a wider ambivalence among clinicians about self-monitoring; as discussed in the Introduction, globally, most app and biosensors are not classified as medical devices and are hence unregulated. Despite some enthusiasm for their role in motivating patients (to exercise more, to lose weight, to track their headaches), there is widespread concern in medical journals that apps and biosensors do not (yet?) produce evidence of bodily states that is reliable or meaningful enough to be used in clinical decision-making (Husain and Spence, 2015; West et al, 2017).

Such reluctance or disinterest is blithely ignored in the promotional materials for apps and biosensors. The webpage of Biodesk (a menopausal-tracking app mentioned in Lippman [2013] as one app that North American family physicians are prescribing), for example, describes the app as a 'medical device', stating that the graphs it produces (using digital diary input from users) can be used by physicians – without any face-to-face consultation – to diagnose and prescribe treatments for menopausal symptoms:

> Biodesk has many useful features making it a unique hormone tracking *medical app* for iPad. It has features of graphing and emailing. With Biodesk you don't need to squander time on taking appointments and waiting outside your specialist's office. Just track your symptoms, get a graph and email it to your specialist. Through graph reports your specialist can analyze your case and make adjustments in therapy accordingly. (Biodesk, 2018, emphasis in original)

These claims suggest that biosensing practices might shift the thresholds of the clinical space by more or less adeptly negotiating, even avoiding, the hurdles of regulation. While possibly unrealistic in practice, they illustrate the centrality of questions of regulation to biosensing and show that prevalent logics of biosensing articulate particular imaginaries of freedom. These are culturally specific and may have more resonance in the US context than in the UK (see Hesse et al, 2005; Nissenbaum and Patterson, 2016; Torous and Roberts, 2017). Our UK panel were keen, in contrast, that the NHS play a key role in regulating biosensing devices and related services, suggesting a kitemark system to facilitate citizens' trust in these (Living Data Research Group, 2013; Mort et al, 2016).

Women's use of fertility biosensing

The question as to whether or not ovulation biosensors and/ or menstrual apps are useful to people trying to become pregnant was, as noted in Box 1.1, central to Wilkinson's study.

In lengthy one-to-one interviews with 27 heterosexual cis-women who were pregnant, had recently given birth or were trying to become pregnant, Wilkinson found that ovulation monitoring provided many women with a meaningful conception-related activity and focus while they were hoping to become pregnant but were not in active fertility treatment. In this sense, even though they may be of little interest to GPs or fertility specialists, results from fertility monitoring arguably become part of a biomedicalised trajectory from a time of 'trying to conceive' through to either prenatal services (if pregnancy occurs) or infertility services. Here, biosensors shape individuals' (often deeply distressing) move from 'the normal' to 'the pathological' in terms of their fertility. Local context matters a lot in these moves: in the UK, it can take more than 12 months for people to access NHS fertility services, which are free at the point of access for a limited number of cycles. Ovulation biosensors (ranging from simple 'pee on a stick' or 'spit in a tube' devices through to more expensive worn thermometers and associated digital technologies), Wilkinson argues, thus populate a highly affectively charged temporal zone along contemporary 'conceptive trails'. Helping those wishing to become pregnant to learn to calibrate their menstrual and ovulatory cycles in ways aligned with biomedical understandings of reproductive bodies, however, the devices prepare users for engagement with assisted conception discourses and biomedical practices such as ovarian stimulation, egg collection and IVF if conception does not occur through intercourse or self-insemination. This is what we refer to as biosensing's 'pre-clinical departure zone'.

During her study, Wilkinson spoke with doctors working in a General Practice that was offering patients ovulation biosensors as part of an informal trial to see if self-monitoring could increase their chance of pregnancy while they were waiting to be offered IVF or related specialist fertility treatment.

These clinicians stated that the biosensing device turned out to be of little help to women and expressed concerns that the remote 'fertility experts' involved in the chosen programme had recommended that users either ask their doctors for Clomid (an ovarian-stimulating medication) or buy it directly online. (Clearly, this advice was intended for North American users; in the UK, such advice is considered unethical.) In more than one case, the 'experts' had also suggested, based solely on her body temperature data, that the user had become pregnant and miscarried. As Wilkinson (2016) found in her interviews with women users, this kind of 'information' and advice can cause a lot of distress to those trying to conceive.

It seems to us that fertility biosensors were being trialled in this General Practice largely as a form of demand management, a way to help those experiencing difficulties conceiving tolerate the challenges of waiting for NHS services to become available to them. As mentioned earlier, it is also important to remember that demonstrating whether or not one ovulates is a key element in accessing fertility services in the UK. While patients may have used ovulation monitors for months, if not years, before accessing reproductive medicine, they will, as the GP stated during the citizens' panel, still be required to take a one-off hormonal test to answer this question. Tracking one's own ovulation might be a reassuring activity for people approaching this formal test, but it cannot replace this biomedical 'hurdle'. 'Knowing' that one ovulates can also constitute a kind of partial fertility (Franklin and Roberts, 2006), helping those undertaking it to adjust to a burgeoning sense of infertility (or a growing challenge to their long-held sense of fertility) that occurs as repeated attempts to become pregnant fail. In other national contexts, using ovulation biosensors will play a different role in 'conceptive trails'. One of Epstein et al's (2017: 17) North American participants reports, for example, that her fertility clinicians were interested in her menstrual tracking data as long as she summarised it in a spreadsheet. In a system in which assisted conception services are privately purchased, there are different hurdles to jump and the time frame of conceptive trails can be quite different to a publicly funded system.

Across the developed world, people who want to become pregnant seem to be willing to spend money on fertility biosensing devices; as noted earlier, there are thought to be millions of current users of fertility-monitoring devices and apps. As feminist scholars have shown, since the development of IVF in the 1980s, cis-women have been subjected to new variations of cultural discourses of risk and responsibility around pregnancy and reproduction (Franklin, 1997; Throsby, 2004; McNeil, 2007). Public discourses, such as those in newspapers, magazines and online sources, consistently blame women for 'leaving it too late' to try to get pregnant and/or for prioritising careers over reproduction. Due to their ubiquity and strength, one could argue that these discourses are subjectifying in the Foucauldian sense (Foucault, 1988); in the current age, 'women' come into being, in part, through engagement with them. Wilkinson found, for example, that many of the participants in her study felt that pregnancy was both difficult to achieve and very precious (see also Throsby, 2004; Franklin and Roberts, 2006). Not becoming pregnant quickly when 'trying to conceive' was thus a highly fraught experience, during which women could easily conjure a variety of self-blaming discourses, as well as a plethora of reparative actions (from healthy eating and increasing physical fitness, to giving up alcohol and trying to improve their sexual lives with their partners). Purchasing and using ovulation monitors has, we suggest, become one of these 'easy-to-take' (but nonetheless difficult to live with) subjectifying actions, issues of affordability notwithstanding. Needless to say, given rising rates of difficulty in conception globally, manufacturers of fertility biosensors stand to make significant profits from these contemporary discourses of risk, self-blame and responsibility.

The 'new fertility' is big business, a valuable part of what Adele Clarke et al (2010) call the 'biomedical–industrial complex'.

Is fertility tracking feminist biosensing?

Feminist theorists and activists have had a long and complex involvement with discourses of reproduction and (in)fertility (Franklin, 2013). At least since the publication of the women's health movement encyclopaedia, *Our Bodies, Ourselves*, in the early 1980s, feminists have advocated that women educate themselves to understand their reproductive bodies both in intimate and personal and in scientific and biomedical ways. Alongside cervical self-examination, coming to know 'ovulation' is an iconic example of such tasks. For 1980s' North American feminists, this involved both temperature taking and recording, and the analysis and recording of cervical and vaginal fluid. While *Our Bodies, Ourselves* was cautious about using knowledge of one's ovulation as a way to make decisions about contraception (for example, refraining from vaginal intercourse on 'fertile days'), monitoring basal body temperature to come to know ovulation patterns was recommended, at least for those with regular menstrual cycles (Connell-Tatum, 1981: 551).

As noted earlier, these practices of 'coming to know' one's ovulation have rapidly diversified and expanded with the roll-out of new reproductive technologies and the rise in infertility rates across the world. According to Ombelet et al (2008), 8–12 per cent of couples of reproductive age experience infertility. In resource-rich parts of the world, such experience often leads to medical treatments, including ovarian stimulation, IVF, artificial insemination, pre-implantation genetic diagnosis, egg donation and surrogacy. They also sometimes involve 'reproductive tourism' to poorer parts of the world where treatment and services can be accessed more cheaply, outside strict regulatory regimes. In many parts of the developing world, such as Egypt, India, China and parts of Northern (but notably not sub-Saharan) Africa, people with sufficient funds – and this often involves 'catastrophic expenditure'[7] – can also access reproductive medicine, including IVF (Inhorn and Patrizio, 2015).

While the early days of such technologies saw concerted feminist resistance and concern (Franklin, 2013), since the 1990s, feminist theorists and activists have engaged more deeply with the emotional and social difficulties associated with infertility and the possibilities that the so-called 'new reproductive technologies' can offer to those in such situations. Some have celebrated the fact that processes such as IVF can be used to conceive children without heterosexual intercourse, thus opening the door to a wider range of people to become birth parents (Marina et al, 2010; Zeiler and Malmquist, 2014). Combining practices of egg donation, IVF and surrogacy have similarly facilitated some people's access to reproduction outside of heterosexual sex (Bergman et al, 2010). While some feminists continue to express concern about the ways in which reproductive processes are harnessed by science and medicine in these procedures, others argue that the value of such interventions needs to be assessed on an ongoing basis (see, for example, Almeling, 2007).

Neither ovulation monitoring (including menstrual apps and biosensing devices) nor semen-quality or sex-hormone monitoring technologies have come under the same level of feminist scrutiny to date. As domestic, non-interventionist technologies that remain largely in the hands of consumers, it perhaps seems that much less is at stake politically and socially when compared to state-sponsored and regulated (or, indeed, privately funded and unregulated) IVF (or, for that matter, gender transition biomedicine). As noted earlier, such self-tracking also potentially fits into a feminist framing that coming

---

[7] This is defined by economists as 'any out-of-pocket payment that threatens household survival by exceeding 40% of annual non-food expenditures' (Inhorn and Patrizio, 2015: 422).

to know one's body better is empowering, even an ethical or political 'good'. In recent years, however, there have been some critical discussions emerging in online and research articles, particularly about menstrual and ovulation tracking. Critics have focused on the ways in which normative ideas of sex, sexuality, gender and reproduction are built into such technologies and apps. In an article published in *Culture, Health and Sexuality*, for example, a group of the current authors argued that ovulation biosensing discourses assume and promote a heteronormative model of reproductive sex, in which sexual intercourse is initiated by men and women's sexual desires (including those relating to the desire to conceive) ideally remain unspoken (Wilkinson et al, 2015). Reproductive heterosex, we claimed, is framed as a kind of technologically enhanced romance in which couples are freed from the difficulties of managing infertility, including discussing intercourse 'timing' with one's partner, which are outsourced to the biosensing program (including the device, the distant fertility experts and the related mobile messages that inform users when they are most fertile). These representations are detailed in promotional videos on the product website, and more subtly in the use of icons on the device, such as love hearts to signal sexual intercourse. In a related argument, Epstein et al (2017: 12) show that menstrual-tracking apps articulate normative ideas about both heterosex and sex/gender via the use of pink, sparkles, flowers and euphemistic, 'cutesy' references to sexual intercourse and body parts, reporting that many participants found these patronising, offensive or insulting (although a minority were positive about 'girly' styling) (see also Lupton, 2015).

Importantly, however, the fact that apps and biosensors build in normative figurations of bodies and relations does not preclude their use for non-normative purposes. Tracking flows of sex hormones and related bodily processes (such as menstruation or body hair growth) can also be of great interest to people undergoing gender transition, or for lesbians or single people wishing to use donor sperm to conceive. Apps and biosensing devices can thus become part of a broader contestation of conventional ideas about the relations between sexed bodies and lived gender identity. Indeed, some app designers have already picked up on such use and are orienting their products towards these emerging markets, refraining from conventional gender coding in choice of colours, icon design and language (see, for example, Collins, 2018; Wilson, 2018).

Our (reproductive) bodies, our data?

A different line of contemporary feminist criticism questions the commercialisation of reproduction and the possible uses of ovulation and menstrual data by companies producing apps and biosensors. Analysis discussed in the *British Medical Journal* (McCarthy, 2013) found that a large proportion of health and fitness apps did not have privacy policies or adequate procedures for encrypting users' data. Self-tracking data, traceable back to a particular individual, could often, then, be legally shared with third parties (such as insurance companies) without the user's knowledge or agreement, or, indeed, stolen (for an analysis of the legalities of sharing biosensing data in Europe and the US, and of users' views of risks to their privacy, see Leibenger et al, 2016). Biosensing devices such the Temperature Egg analysed by Wilkinson collect temperature- and ovulation-related data collected via worn devices, reportedly in order to assist 'fertility experts' to understand users' fertility patterns and then to advise when heterosexual intercourse should take place. While individuals' data remain 'strictly confidential' and 'encrypted', it is aggregated with other users' data in order, the manufacturers claim on their website, to build algorithms that are more likely to help their in-house 'fertility experts' to predict a particular user's ovulation and to recognise any undiagnosed fertility problem (such as polycystic ovary syndrome). In an interview with Wilkinson, a senior representative of the Temperature Egg manufacturer said:

> More importantly it has the ability to recalculate and change the algorithm for every patient on an individual basis. And so we do that with having all the data come back to our servers here so when the patient connects they monitor all the data sent via the internet. We receive it here – it's processed in our server as well as online by a team. So we can manually say that a patient has PCOS [polycystic ovary syndrome], she's therefore likely not to have a pattern like someone who doesn't have that condition. And so the system will fit her – an algorithm that is most likely to work for someone with PCOS. But after the first cycle of using it, you will recognise patterns that are seen in a subpopulation of patients with PCOS, which will optimise the algorithm going forward. (Wilkinson, 2014)

In the same way that Fitbit data about steps and sleep can be used to explore wider social patterns of health and activity (as discussed in the Introduction), however, aggregated reproduction-related data might also be used to build claims about fertility more broadly. In *The Guardian*, journalist Moira Weigel (2016) argues that, at the very least, menstrual-tracking apps could collect data on individuals to facilitate the direct marketing of related products (such as tampons and pads), and that using such apps thus assists the commercialisation of reproductive flows:

> "People trying to get pregnant are a very marketable segment," Karen Levy, a professor at Cornell University who focuses on monitoring technologies, told me. Pregnant women start needing things they never needed before: tubs of lotion, prenatal vitamins, diapers. Long-held

brand loyalties come up for grabs, and shopping habits shift. "So advertisers already know something huge about you if they know you are using a fertility app," Levy said. Some users might feel reservations about volunteering so much data, if they understood just how valuable it was, and how it could be used to target them. (Weigel, 2016; see also Levy, 2015)

Knowledge about women's menstrual cycles and their attempts to conceive could, in other words, become valuable information to both relevant commercial and biomedical and public health researchers, and could ultimately be used to accumulate 'biovalue' (Waldby and Cooper, 2010) within contemporary economies of reproduction. Such accumulation is facilitated by the biodigital platformisation of biosensing, through which researchers and corporations gain direct access to billions of 'data points'. Crawford et al (2015: 494) make a related argument, remarking that '[T]he relationship between users, devices and companies is fluctuating, and the full use of the data is always out of sight to the user'. Additionally, they argue that:

[T]he economic value of the data, be it for the wearables company to increase its perceived value as a big data collector or as a set to be traded and sold, is never shared with the users who make up that data set. Neither may users extract or 'delete' their data if they stop using the wearable device. (Crawford et al, 2015: 494)

Some app designers address these criticisms head-on in their promotional materials. On its detailed and complex website and associated blogs and vlogs, the Science and Education Manager of menstrual-tracking app 'Clue', Anna Druet, discusses the issue of data aggregation and sharing, claiming that women and society in general have much to gain from the ways in which their tracking data is used by scientists:

When you track in Clue, you contribute to an unprecedented data set that is forwarding the understanding of female health in a new frontier of health research. We work with top research institutions and clinicians to explore topics with real-world impact – to better understand our bodies and physical mechanisms, explore our cultural and demographic diversity, and to break harmful taboos. (Druet, 2018)

Indeed, on this website and in many other public settings, the Chief Executive Officer of 'Clue', Danish entrepreneur Ida Tin, suggests that 'we' will not have an 'equal world' until women understand more about their reproductive bodies. (Interestingly, in these statements, she tends to revert to gendered language, despite the company's policy to try to avoid it.) In a discussion about the risks of data sharing and data security on the Clue website, for example, she writes:

When you collect data about your health, you have the possibility to take care of your body, be informed, and get care. Your biggest risk is not that your app company gets hacked, but rather that it was founded by people whose ethical choices you might not agree with. That's why you must choose wisely who you share your data with. (Tin, 2018)

Later, she firmly promises, in bold, italics and in stand-alone paragraphs to emphasise, that:

We don't sell your data. Full stop.

and that:

I believe that the benefits of living in an age of data outweigh the risks. (Tin, 2018)

Clue does, she states, 'share data points ... with carefully-selected health researchers' (Tin, 2018), but Tin reminds readers that all such data is anonymised. A list of researchers is available on the website, and includes anthropologists, evolutionary psychologists, biomedical informatics specialists and clinicians interested in sexuality, reproduction, menstruation and contraception (Tin, 2018). Tin also insists that 'we don't make any money from this. We actually spend a lot of resources on these collaborations – data analysts, research coordinators, and so on. So it *costs* us money for us to do them'(2018, emphasis in original). This is an interesting statement – indeed, in the business and financial press, journalists note that it remains unclear how companies like Clue will 'monetise' their work. An article in the *Business Insider Australia*, for example, articulates the kind of dilemma that Tin faces:

> Ask Ida Tin what her goal is, and she struggles to come up with just one. The top of the App Store's health and fitness section would be nice, she says (she's only got to third place before) – or maybe helping every woman on the planet track their reproductive health. (Cook, 2016)[8]

This journalist quotes Tin as stating that she is not willing to sell users' data or to include advertisements in the app. Instead, Tin suggests that Clue might invite users to pay for 'more in-depth data-driven information or health advice' (Cook, 2016) in order to generate revenue. In this scenario, knowledge acquired from the 'secure' data points would be sold back to those who generated them. One also wonders about who would provide the health advice.

---

[8] After establishing Clue in 2013, Tin went on to act as an advisor to Apple in 2015, helping them to correct their astonishing omission of fertility in the first iteration of 'HealthKit', the Apple Watch biosensing platform, through including a period-tracking element in the watch.

Like the manufacturers of other kinds of biosensors (such as Fitbits), then, the makers of ovulation biosensors such as the Temperature Egg and menstrual-tracking apps such as Clue describe the accumulation or aggregation of data flows from individuals' devices as positive opportunities for users. The App Store page for Clue encourages users to 'Track alongside with millions of people for accurate information' (BioWink GmbH, 2018). The meaning of 'alongside' in this context is specific: it refers to the fact that users can compare their data to the norms produced by the aggregated data of other users, and/or use related online interfaces to discuss their data with other users. In her study of the Temperature Egg and the ovulation microscope, Wilkinson found that many users were, at least for certain periods of their 'conceptive trails', engaging in detailed discussion online with other users. In many instances, this was driven by their desire to understand and interpret the somewhat unclear data produced when using the devices. Spitting into the ovulation microscope, for example, is supposed to produce 'ferning patterns' if you are ovulating. Online discussions were filled with women discussing what 'ferning' looks like, what it meant if you seemed to be ovulating but still did not conceive or how one might organise a sexual encounter to be timed with ovulation without humiliating or upsetting one's partner (Wilkinson, 2016). Wilkinson's study, then, showed that women using biosensors in their attempts to conceive do, indeed, 'track alongside ... others'; however, it also demonstrated that such practices were more often associated with uncertainty and confusion than with 'accurate information' or clarity. Discussing one's own biosensing data with others did not always create greater understanding (although it sometimes did), but it did often seem to lead to some of kind of psychosocial relief. Members of online fertility forums reassured each other, swapped information and ideas, and managed to find the humour in some of the difficulties associated with the hurdles that they were encountering along their conceptive trails.

It is interesting to note the limits of such sharing, however. At no point did these online conversations turn towards the kinds of political questions that were (and remain) a constitutive element of feminist Women's Health Movements' attempts to take back control of their reproductive bodies and to understand the real causes of ill health, including infertility; participants were not trying to challenge conventional biomedical understandings of sexed/gendered bodies. Neither do online discussions of ovulation monitoring among heterosexual cis-women – as studied by Wilkinson – delve into the causes of decline in human reproductive function, the rise of infertility or the politics of stratified access to biomedical fertility services.

In notable contrast, online discussions of and blogs about menstrual tracking produced by gender-queer, agender and/ or trans people are regularly peppered with critical comments about the ways in which biosensing technologies and related apps figure sex/gender and sexuality. In a vlog about the 'Period and Health Tracker' Clue, for example, YouTuber ChandlerNWilson (Wilson, 2018) produces a sharp critique of the way in which most menstrual-tracking apps assume that a menstruating person is a woman. Apparently paid to do so (although this is not stated on the vlog) (Bell, 2018), Wilson promotes Clue's app for resisting this conflation and making virtual and physical space for menstruating men and gender-queer others. In this discourse, and similar others, the politics of sex/gender formations and sexual norms, and their problematic enactments in contemporary biomedicine, are central to discussions of the usefulness of self-tracking. As both Wilson's vlog and a related article on the Clue website note (Bell, 2018), knowing when one is likely to menstruate can be hugely important to people living as men in their social milieus: being caught short without sanitary products can produce socially awkward scenarios. Tracking menstruation for those taking testosterone can also provide important feedback on the body's hormonal changes (over time, taking testosterone should lead to the cessation of menstruation). Biomedical knowledge about gender transition remains in development, so the online sharing of physical and other experiences is hugely important to the formation of usable knowledge about hormonal experiences.

Epstein et al (2017: 14) recommend that menstrual apps are designed for customisation, reporting that users are keen to have flexible interfaces that are discreet and malleable to their own situation (for example, whether or not they have sexual intercourse, whether they are trying to pregnant, and whether they identify as men, women or something else). This finding chimes with our earlier work on telecare devices (discussed in Chapter 4) in which we also recommend that devices remain open to user customisation, arguing that such designs are more ethical (Mort et al, 2013). Interestingly, Epstein et al (2017: 16) also recommend that menstrual apps have the capacity to search for correlations with other self-tracking data such as that relating to physical activity or mood. Users in their study were keen to explore interactions between their menstrual cycles and other physical and emotional experiences. This finding also resonates with Nafus's (2016a) arguments that biosensing data is most interesting to users when they can become part of small-scale life experiments, testing connections across previously poorly connected life events.

Wilkinson's study demonstrates that using fertility biosensors to track ovulation is not enough to ensure participation in critical conversations about reproductive bodies. Knowing more about ovulation and menstruation, in other words, is not sufficient for critical narratives to arise. 'Data' – in the form of information about hormonal flows or temperature – is too hygienic, too divorced from biopsychosocial embodiment to provide insight, even when shared with 'millions of other users'. This is not to say, however, that such data might not have an important part to play in critical projects of knowledge creation and contestation. Learning more about patterns of ovulation and menstruation across millions of users – when correlated with other data pertaining to life experience and geographical, social and historical location, for example – could be highly informative for political health-related projects.

The problem for users of corporate biosensing systems, however, is that they are not able to access the aggregated data – such information is reserved for particular researchers and insurance or other companies, who may or may not have liberatory goals. As Crawford et al (2015: 494) argue, in most apps and systems, users can only access a thin slice of data:

> The body is tracked, documented and rendered meaningful through a device that records a wealth of data for the parent company, third parties and possibly insurers and employers, and only a small fraction of the potential and value of this data is returned to the user. Beyond the clear economic disparity, companies like Jawbone and Fitbit get to see aggregated data: the patterns of activity (and inactivity) across geography, class and gender among many other possible categories. This god's eye view offers a significant and politically charged perspective – yet the user only gets to see their individual behavior compared to a norm, a speck in the larger sea of data.

Additionally, as Crawford et al (2015: 494) argue, '[U]sers of wearables are told very little about the cultural and scientific assumptions that undergird notions of the normal user, and they are simply placed in percentiles that lack any transparency in their construction or use'.

Even if users could access relevant databases, as can selected researchers and companies, then many other forms of data and knowledge would, in our view, be needed to produce the kinds of outcomes that feminists and other critical scholars and activists desire. Due to this, we would strongly contest Ida Tin's claim that self-tracking will ultimately create an 'equal world'; indeed, without adequate political and intellectual engagement, it could very easily contribute to producing a much less equal one.

Critical experiments in fertility biosensor design

Some researchers try to bring a more critical approach to fertility biosensor design. In a PhD project at the University of Copenhagen, for example, Sarah Homewood has designed an ambient light that projects different colours into a room of the user's house according to the stage of their menstrual cycle, using data gleaned from a menstrual-tracking phone app. This project attempts to address taboos around menstruation that remain despite the flourishing of tracking apps, taking an individual's data and making it visible (via colour) in their home, so that those living with them can 'know' what stage of the cycle they are experiencing. Significantly, the project also explores the possible dissonance between an individual's experience of their bodies and moods, and biomedical ideas about what is 'supposed' to happen at each stage of the menstrual cycle. The colours of the ambient light represent 'typical' moods at various points in a conventional cycle: heightened irritability just before menstruation and increased sexual desire at mid-cycle, for example. Projecting these norms onto the ceiling, Homewood's (2018) 'Ambient cycle' technology is meant to give space for users to challenge these representations by comparing how they 'really' feel to the colours in the room.

A different experimental biosensing project, from researchers at Newcastle University in the UK, intentionally cites the early work of Women's Health Movements on vaginal phobia and women's lack of knowledge about their physical bodies. Famously, in the 1970s and 1980s, groups of North American feminists developed practices of gynaecological self-examination in groups in order to address these serious concerns. Using technologies of modern medicine (the speculum) alongside more domestic and home-made technologies (hand mirrors and sometimes flexible tubing), cis-women taught each other how to see and observe their genitals and reproductive anatomy (most importantly, the cervix). The Newcastle Labella project involves biosensing underwear linked to a mobile phone app. The underwear records images of the wearer's genitals, which are then displayed onscreen framed by an image of a Snow White-style mirror. Real-time video data can help users to practice pelvic fitness – the app includes coached sessions of pelvic floor exercises aimed to develop a 'nuanced understanding of pelvic muscle structure' and in that way to come to 'know', both visually and via sensation, their reproductive bodies better.

A third example, designed by students at Wellesley College, Massachusetts, notes the typical 'feminisation' of menstrual apps and biosensing systems discussed earlier. The counter-design – the Crimson Wave – involves an armband thermometer worn at night to collect basal body temperature and a connected smart mirror, the frame of which changes colour according to the stage of the menstrual cycle that the user's temperature data indicates they are in. This device is intended to take the labour out of using standard menstrual apps (no manual input of data is needed) and to allow users to assess their hormonal status at a glance in the mirror. Deliberately simple, the Crimson Wave does not give any additional advice or information (Flemings et al, 2018) and makes no attempts to connect users in any way.

In her analysis of the 1980s' North American Women's Health Movements' practices of cervical self-examination, Donna Haraway (1997: 193) argues that these ran the risk of naively assuming that 'seeing' amounts to critical knowledge. However, as Michelle Murphy (2012) demonstrates, these practices arose from and were a pivotal part of a wider political movement aimed at challenging patriarchal accounts of the discursive and material control of women's bodies. Women's understanding of their cervixes, for example, depended on comparison with others, on group discussion and participation, and on shared documentation through drawing, photography and video (Murphy, 2012). The critical fertility biosensing projects discussed earlier pick up on only some elements of this history and fail to understand or capture the collective aspects of female bodily self-examination, what Murphy (2012), developing Haraway's (1997) work on the 'modest witness' of modern science, calls 'immodest witnessing'. Viewed through a feminist technoscience studies lens, these critical biosensing projects highlight the significant tensions between individual bodily experiences (collected over time), aggregated data from many individual users and biomedical knowledge and norms. Such tensions are precisely the place where Women's Health Movements developed an alternative set of data collection practices in order to build feminist knowledge about bodies, sex/gender and reproduction. Despite their shortcomings, the explicit connections to feminist histories of body tracking and health politics, and the attempt to explore the limits of self-tracking and biosensing (rather than to accept their data as accurate or 'true' representations of bodies), render such experiments notably different from corporate technologies such as the Apple Watch or Clue (despite the latter's vague referencing of liberal feminist ideals). As Rachel Sanders (2017: 38) argues in relation to weight and exercise apps and biosensors, it is important to note that while self-monitoring can increase individuals' level of knowledge about their bodies, which can be experienced as empowering, such practices can simultaneously 'serve the convergent interests of biopower and gender retrenchment'.

Conclusions

Biosensing is becoming part of the formation of contemporary sexed/gendered bodies and the ways in which we understand human reproduction to occur. What can we learn from earlier feminist research on new reproductive technologies and from recent debates and experiments around fertility and hormonal tracking? First, framing biosensing as a simple colonisation of bodies or an elaborate exercise in neoliberal self-governance is a rather limiting approach that fails to recognise either individuals' or groups' strong attachments to related practices and devices. Second, biosensing may have value for critical health and life projects. This is not, clearly, to say that biosensing of any sort should simply be celebrated as a positive form of grass-roots knowledge production.

Biosensing should, we suggest, be understood as part of highly complex biomedical and social media platforms that require careful and detailed social-scientific analysis. Contemporary biosensing negotiates shifting thresholds between clinical and other forms of expertise, taking place in mediated forms that render experience comparable, exchangeable and commodifiable in previously impossible ways. A range of biomedical and clinical processes, including those pertaining to assisted conception, gender transition and the menopause, may change in the light of the platformisation of fertility and hormonal biosensing – if such biosensing reshapes the contours of reproduction and sex/gender, then people may arrive in clinics at different times of their lives, with newly articulated goals and with a very different sense of their life course.

Fertility biosensors articulate bodies in particular ways and typically rely on highly conventional accounts of sex/gender, sexuality and reproduction in their design. As we have argued, however, this reliance does not preclude their use for non-normative and/or critical projects. Fertility biosensors, in other words, provide a clear example of the ways in which biosensors more broadly readily reaffirm conventional distinctions between the normal and the pathological, but also provide examples of the ways in which they can do something quite different if used in concert with other forms of critical engagement.

2

Biosensing Stress

Since the 1970s, adult citizens of the Global North have been encouraged to learn to notice when they are physiologically stressed, and to hone skills to alleviate stress in the name of improving their mental and physical health, their social relationships, and their productivity at work. Today, many technology companies offer devices and/or apps to assist users to develop such knowledge and skills. These range from apps to teach stress recognition and relaxation techniques (such as Fitbit's and Apple Watch's breathing apps), through to worn heart-rate variability or skin conductivity sensors, and saliva and blood sampling kits to send off to laboratories to measure levels of so-called 'stress hormones'. 'Stress', although remaining complex and elusive as a scientific phenomenon and experience, is rapidly becoming rearticulated through biosensing devices and platforms in ways that could have serious repercussions for how we live, including, importantly, how adults and children are monitored and assessed by remote others, such as employers, parents, teachers, social and corrective services officials, and health insurance companies.

The assessment of stress via biosensing blends culturally and historically specific experiences of, ideas about and practices to ameliorate physical and psychological discomfort. Knowledges and practices developed in Eastern traditions, including yoga, meditation and mindfulness, are blended with a body of Western scientific work that dates back more than 100 years. Developed most notably by Hungarian-Canadian scientist Hans Selye (1907–82) from the 1930s to the 1970s, this scientific work elaborated the late 19th-/early 20th-century notions of 'internal chemical environments' and 'homeostasis' posited by French physiologist Claude Bernard (1818–78) and North American Walter Cannon (1871–1945). As detailed later, from the 1970s, Selye's theories about the role of hormones in maintaining homeostasis, and his notions of 'good' and 'bad' stress, widely infiltrated public and clinical discourse with a narrative of 'balance' that can be disrupted by external stimuli such as overwork, interpersonal difficulties and major life events. This narrative also has important resonance with Chinese and other Eastern understandings of physical and mental health that were widely promulgated in the US, UK and Europe in the 1980s (Franklin et al, 2000; Jackson, 2013: 258). Used widely in relevant 'self-health' literatures (Franklin et al, 2000) as both a verb and a noun, 'balance' has become something for individuals to strive for in order to maximise health and life chances and even to be happy. In emerging biosensing discourses, this 'balance' is parsed at a physiological level, in terms of breathing and/or heart-rate variability, galvanic skin conductivity, and/or levels and patterns of stress hormones.

Following Selye, who famously distinguished between 'stress' (the physiological experience) and 'stressors' (factors that cause stress), popular accounts (including self-help books, online guides and leaflets) describe individuals as having personal responses to stressors that involve greater or lesser physiological changes, which, in turn, are associated with long-term harms such as heart disease and cancer. In a popular book published as part of the highly successful 'Teach Yourself' series, entitled *Managing stress*, for example, Looker and Gregson (2003 [1997]: 34, emphasis in original) write:

The differences in the extent of activation of the stress response within or beyond the normal zone of the stress balance depend on how you view or interpret situations around you and on how you feel about those situations.

This means that stress is not in the environment but is a *state within you*. The way in which you transact with the environment determines how much and what type of stress you create for yourself.

In this discourse, keeping one's stress in 'balance' becomes a personal responsibility precisely because the stress is 'a state within you' and not an external force, and is dependent on how 'you transact with the environment'. Configured as an internal bodily state, stress is ripe for biosensing. Importantly, these discourses do not contend that one's reactions to stressors are somehow only biological. Life experiences matter, as do genes and other physical factors:

> Our interpretation of the nature of the demand and how well we feel able to cope with it depends on our experience of past events, our beliefs, attitudes, expectations and needs. These in turn depend on our genetic inheritance, personality, education, upbringing, age, sex and general state of health. (Looker and Gregson, 2003 [1997]: 34)

Nonetheless, in such literatures, the responsibility lies with individuals to manage their own reactions – to 'teach yourself' how to manage stress – and this shift towards individual responsibility resonates strongly with contemporary self-monitoring discourses and practices. Biosensing stress, then, fits well into the second column of Table 0.1 (see Introduction): it is a practice of 'self-health' that remains (as yet) rather distant from clinical medicine. However, as Table 0.1 notes, and we discuss in greater detail later, results from stress testing may also be of interest to others beyond the individual tester: the US military, for example, uses heart-rate monitors to record stress levels in troops, while corporate finance companies also ask employees to wear devices in order to become aware when they are 'in the zone' and when they are too stressed to work effectively.

Box 2.1: Living with cortisol

By Celia Roberts and Adrian Mackenzie

The argument in this chapter is underpinned by the experience of Roberts and Mackenzie in the British adoption field, an experience that we have recently begun to document and draw upon in academic publications and presentations (Roberts, 2016; Mackenzie and Roberts, 2017). Through more than ten years of 'observant participation', we have acquired a rich, embodied experience of contemporary discourses that describe the long-term biopsychosocial legacies of early life trauma, disruption and/or loss, and advise adoptive parents how to help children with these backgrounds. Alongside our adoptive-parent friends, we have been trained, in multiple venues ranging from one-to-one sessions with psychotherapists and clinical psychologists, through small groups with social workers, to large conference venues with hundreds of parents or professionals, to understand the neuroscience of stress and trauma. We have also frequently become lay educators ourselves in this field: explaining our children's difficulties to school teachers, leaders of extracurricular activity groups and other parents, and offering strategies and advice on how to best to help everyone manage better. We have provided interviews for newspapers and radio, appeared in documentary films for relevant charities, and participated in long-term informal and formal support groups.

In all of these encounters, we have listened carefully (and where appropriate taken detailed notes), collected printed and other materials, asked questions of our teachers, and discussed endlessly with each other and friends and colleagues (including Maggie Mort) to try to make critical and practical sense of the discourses presented to and by us. We have read widely in the field, exploring both the advice literature for parents and books for children, and more technical scientific and biomedical papers. Most importantly, perhaps, for own understanding, we have also tried to parent our children in ways that align with this knowledge. Such parenting, we have discovered, is an endlessly challenging experiment as regards both our sense of who we are and what it means to be a parent, and what a childhood 'should' look like. 'Therapeutic' or 'brain-based' parenting (Hughes and Baylin, 2012) is an energetic 'journey' of trial and error in which we are faced time and again with frustration, even despair, but also surprise and joy.

In our academic and other public writing and talking, we strive to always protect our children's privacy. We do not discuss any particular difficulties or provide any identifying details. We ask readers and listeners to take us at face value when we say things are hard sometimes. If people want examples of what this means, there are plenty of published accounts, including American psychotherapist Daniel Hughes's (1998) *Building the bonds of attachment* and British adoptive mother

Sally Donovan's (2013) *No matter what: An adoptive family's story of hope, love and healing*, as well as many excellent blogs.

In the contemporary adoptive scene, as we show elsewhere (Mackenzie and Roberts, 2017), neuroscience is prominent. Parents are encouraged to understand themselves and their children as 'embrained' and to come to read behaviour (actions and words), feelings and bodily symptoms (pain, nausea, enuresis, constipation, jitteriness and so on) as connected to brain states. 'Stress' and, more specifically, 'distress' are figured as profoundly embodied echoes of early life experience. *The Connected Child*, a book 'for parents who have welcomed children: from other countries and cultures; from troubled backgrounds; with special behavioural or emotional needs', provides a typical example (Purvis et al, 2007). Written by three North American psychologists specialising in child development, the book advises parents to employ a toolkit of strategies to help their children feel safe (that is, to stop them feeling highly distressed and acting in potentially dangerous ways). These range from controlling the timbre of their voices and speaking simply and repeating themselves, through to drawing up visual charts of each day's activities and engaging in various forms of therapeutic play.

Purvis et al (2007: 53, emphasis added) take readers to the physiology of stress:

Reducing Stress Improves Behavior

Cortisol is a hormone that is activated by and responds to stress. Cortisol levels normally rise and fall at varying times of the day, but when children have too little or too much cortisol in their bodies over an extended period, it can cause serious problems.

By helping your child feel safe, making his or her world more predictable, and teaching better coping skills, *you can actually optimize cortisol levels and allow your child's brain to work better*.

Two figurations are evident here. First, cortisol appears as something to be worked on, even 'optimised', in the name of health and happiness. Second, and this is hinted at rather than explained, cortisol is something that both indexes and *causes* 'serious problems'. As we have argued elsewhere, this turn to cortisol and brains both as explanatory device and something to work on is ubiquitous in contemporary adoptive parenting training. Coming to understand early life trauma today involves engaging with research on neuroendocrinology and brain function – not, importantly, in order to medicate, but to facilitate compassion and to develop adults' and children's capacity to live differently with emotional distress.

What is stress?

Selye's ground-breaking research on rodents in the 1930s–60s explored the physiological effects of external stressors on individual animals. Building on Cannon's and Bernard's exploration of what later came to be known as hormonal flows, Selye articulated an antagonistic, bipartite physiological autonomic nervous system in which the activities of the parasympathetic nervous system (which conserves energy and tends to decrease activity and create relaxation) and the sympathetic nervous system (which causes arousal so that energy can be expended for survival) are in tension (Jackson, 2013). In Selye's model, particular hormones and neurotransmitters are associated with reactions to stressors via both the sympathetic nervous system and the hypothalamic–pituitary–adrenal (HPA) axis. The three key biochemical actors in this model – all of which derive from the adrenal glands, situated above the kidneys – are adrenaline, noradrenaline and cortisol. 'Adrenal' means 'from the kidneys' and 'cortis' means from 'bark' or outer shell. Cortisol is produced on the outer parts of the adrenal glands – the adrenal cortex – and the other two from the adrenal medulla, the inner part of the gland. All of these are produced in response to signals sent from the pituitary gland stimulated by the hypothalamus (both brain structures are central to endocrine flows of all kinds, almost all of which work in negative feedback systems to maintain what Cannon [1963] called homeostasis).

According to Selye, noradrenaline prepares the body to fight, while adrenaline prepares the body to run away. Cortisol, in contrast, prepares the body to shut down in situations of threat. These three key responses are parsed as 'fight, flight or freeze'. Adrenaline and noradrenaline are important in situations of immediate threat, and lead to quick action. Triggered by stressors, increases in adrenaline or noradrenaline have an excitatory effect on the body, overwhelming the parasympathetic system (which is oriented towards calmness). Cortisol flows are more likely, as discussed later, to be significantly altered in situations of more enduring stressors, helping the body to maintain itself in longer-term demanding conditions. Cortisol prepares the body to survive attack by mobilising glucose, reducing allergic responses, reducing inflammation and promoting wound healing, and also sensitises organs to adrenaline and noradrenaline.

Importantly, Selye and others following his model point out that a degree of stress is valuable and even pleasurable – they call this 'eustress'. Eustress is enlivening and helps us to get on with life. Too much stress, in contrast, becomes 'distress'. Individuals, the self-help literature argues, should learn to distinguish the two.[1] In popular guidance based on the Selyian model, individuals are advised to learn how to recognise physical signs of stress. Citizens are figured as generally unaware of these and requiring training to be able to feel and know them: because they are so common, they become 'normal'. As Looker and Gregson (2003 [1997]: 63, emphasis in original) write:

> Most people do not usually associate these signs with distress and secondly, many people are under distress so much of the time that these activities have become habitual and are therefore never associated with distress. This raises an important point. *We must all learn to listen to our body and to read and take notice of the messages it is sending.*

The physical signs of stress are multiple and involve a wide range of bodily organs and systems: like all hormonal actors, cortisol, adrenaline and noradrenaline flow throughout the body with multiple effects. While adrenaline and noradrenaline remain rather constant in the body unless a particular event occurs, cortisol has daily (diurnal) patterns of ebb and flow, with cortisol levels typically highest on waking and declining over the day. 'Signs' of

---

[1] Although still widely taught and promulgated, this understanding of a bipartite autonomic nervous system (sympathetic versus parasympathetic) is today contested by other scientists, most prominently, perhaps, North American neuropsychiatrist Stephen Porges (2011).

increased stress include increased heart-rate variability, atypical skin conductivity, the suppression of immune responses, goose pimples and stomach aches, increased micturition and diarrhoea, pupil dilation, clenched jaws, and atypically acute hearing. Many of these symptoms are easy enough to feel once one attends to them – others less so – but all involve developing awareness and knowledge of typically involuntary physiological processes.

Paying attention to breathing, for example, has been a core task in the self-health stress literature since the 1970s. Learning to breathe deeply and regularly, that is 'correctly', is important, Looker and Gregson (2003 [1997]: 130) argue. Contemporary devices combine biosensors and apps to train users in this skill. The Fitbit, for example, offers a visually simple breathing animation in which users are encouraged to spend two or five minutes matching their breathing pattern to an animated graphic of a small circle moving in and out. These sessions are 'individualised': Fitbit's wrist biosensor measures the user's heart rate and uses animated sparkles in its display to indicate that the user is following the animation properly and thus reducing their heart rate (Fitbit, 2018). At the end of this sequence, the device rewards users with written praise and showers of animated fireworks. Attending to breathing is also part of many Eastern bodily practices, most notably, Buddhist meditation, and many contemporary biosensors borrow language from these traditions to explain why breathing can help to reduce stress. The Apple Watch's Breathe app, for example, 'guides you through a series of deep breaths and … reminds you to take time to breath everyday' (Apple Inc, 2018). Using this app, Apple Watch wearers can log how many 'mindful minutes' they accumulate over a period of time, and view a graph of this pattern. Both the Fitbit and Apple Watch also measure heart rate, and encourage users to notice how their heart rate changes after a session of guided breathing. How users should connect this back to a felt experience of stress is less clear.

Before the era of contemporary biosensors, Looker and Gregson (2003 [1997]) suggested using 'biofeedback' techniques – a key precursor of biosensing – to measure the more elusive physiological processes associated with stress, such as galvanic skin response (sweatiness). Specifically, they advised the use of adhesive 'biodots' that, stuck to the skin, change colour when skin temperature shifts (Looker and Gregson, 2003 [1997]: 134–5). Importantly, the use of biodots was recommended only alongside a range of more cognitive forms of self-assessment, organised through questionnaires about lifestyle, health habits and typical reactions to daily situations. Knowing one's skin temperature is of little use in this approach unless one also knows what one tends to find stressful and whether or not one has a 'Type A' personality (see Jackson, 2013: 208–9). In 1977, two British psychologists developed the 'Stress Watch' based on biofeedback models. This watch was intended to help stressed individuals to monitor their stress response 'at a glance' and thus 'thrive on [positive] stress' (Jackson, 2013: 222–3).

In 2018, consumers can purchase a much wider range of devices and tests to measure physiological signs of stress. Many of these look like watches or jewellery. The Moodmetric ring, for example, is a Finnish-designed 'mood' ring that, like the biodots, measures galvanic skin response over time. Like most contemporary biosensors, in addition to real-time display (in this case, through colour change), this device is linked to an app that records and then charts one's changing stress levels over time. Heart-rate variability (the gap between heartbeats while you are resting) – another sign of stress – can also be measured with watch-like devices, linked to mobile phone apps that record and represent changes over time. Such devices are frequently used by athletes to measure cardiac fitness, explaining, perhaps, their greater ubiquity. Consumers are encouraged to 'kill two birds with one stone' through such devices: monitoring their physical fitness and their stress levels (see, for example, Laidler, 2017). Other devices measure breathing rate through clothing – the Vitali bra is one example (Maslakovic, 2017) – while others measure brain activity (via electroencephalography). The latter can, it is claimed, be life-changing devices for people with epilepsy (Empatica Inc, 2018).

At the time of writing, it is not possible, either in clinics or outside them, to measure the hormones associated with stress – cortisol, adrenaline and noradrenaline – in a continuous way. Nor is it possible to measure them in one-off occasions at home (this is in contrast to various sex hormones, which can be measured in one-off, domestic tests, such as the ovulation microscope discussed in Chapter 1). Measurements of stress hormones are derived from blood or saliva samples that must be sent to laboratories, as in the direct-to-consumer genetic testing discussed in Chapter 3. Unlike genetic testing, however, the results of one-off tests provide scant information – by their very nature, hormones shift over time and vary across individuals. One would need to engage in regular testing – as do consumers of blood glucose testing, for example – to get a sense of how one's hormonal flows are affected by stress.

This fact does not deter companies from offering one-off tests of cortisol and/or 'adrenal function', and thus articulating the cultural logic of biosensing that promotes the value of knowing one's physical data. Advertising for such tests, unsurprisingly, downplays (or even fails to mention) cortisol's diurnal and longer fluctuations. Consumers looking to 'improve their sports performance' and willing to spend £39 on a blood test by forthwithlife.co.uk, for example, will receive just one measure of (waking) cortisol levels, from which they are told that they will be able to 'check your adrenal function, check whether your body may be under too much stress and check whether you may be overtraining' (Forth, 2018a). Others willing to spend up to £79 per test several times a year can 'subscribe' to a programme of repeated tests of up to 20 different biomarkers to come to understand their body's health. 'Rather than a short-term snapshot', the website promises:

> our subscription route enables you to build your own unique biomarker profile giving you long-term insight into your health. Through on–going testing you can track how

your body is responding to changes in your lifestyle either through diet or exercise. This means you can spot potential areas for improvement before they become problems, so you can enjoy a healthier, fitter, stronger life. (Forth, 2018b)

Such sites articulate a Selyian understanding of hormonal balance and 'stress load' (Forth, 2018c). The webpage of Smart Nutrition, a company offering saliva cortisol testing, for example, states that:

Sometimes in periods of long-term or severe mental or physical stress these glands can go into overdrive. If this occurs for too long or too often then the adrenals later become exhausted. When this happens, the hormonal levels of Cortisol, DHEA [a related adrenal hormone] in the bloodstream become imbalanced. (Smart Nutrition, 2018)

'Having balanced stress hormones', the text insists (in bold font), 'is particularly important' because they:

Maintain emotional and physical energy
Strengthen the immune system against colds, coughs, flu and possibly more serious illness
Improve metabolism, help reduce fat storage, and control appetite
Slow down the aging process, decrease PMS [premenstrual syndrome] and menstrual difficulties
Aid dietary protein synthesis – helping mood
Prevent osteoporosis
Maintain healthy blood pressure levels
Lower LDL [low-density lipoprotein] 'bad' cholesterol levels. (Smart Nutrition, 2018)

Tests cost £85 and consumers are offered a report like that shown in Figure 2.1. Although the laboratory leader states that he 'still finds the test clinically significant', no advice is offered as to how 'patients' are supposed to work with the information obtained. 'Patients' are advised to take their results to clinicians, but it remains unclear as to what is meant to be demonstrated by one's 'adrenal stress profile'. These offerings and advice, we argue, articulate a contemporary biosensing logic that assumes – with little or no evidence – that such data will be of interest and value to clinicians and individuals in health assessments and decision-making. These websites describe a world that, as we argued in Chapter 1, remains quite remote from contemporary arrangements constituting general and specialist medical practices.

Figure 2.1: Screenshot of a sample 'adrenal stress profile' sent to test purchasers

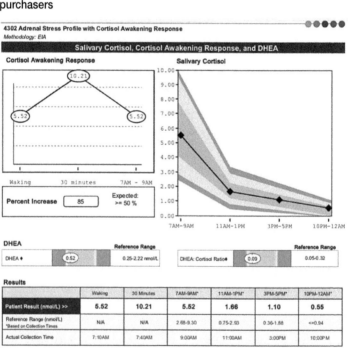

Source: With permission of Genova Diagnostics UK; Peace-Brewer (2009)

Configuring stress

Seylian talk of 'balance' and 'load', and the recognition that stress can be positive and negative, are ubiquitous in stress biosensing discourses. The website for the Moodmetric ring, for example, advises consumers to:

> Find the balance between work and free time – excitement, stress and recovery are all part of a good life. Stress is a natural reaction to a situation that requires adaptation. Right amount of stress keeps us active, motivated and enthusiastic. Demands of work, family, hobbies and activities summing up to a big load can go unnoticed. The body does not know whether stress is positive or negative. Recovery is necessary also when things are great! (See: www.moodmetric.com/)

Here, both bodies and people are figured as ignorant: consumers do not know if they are stressed, and bodies cannot tell the difference between eustress and distress. Like the biodot users of the 1990s, then, those wearing Moodmetric rings are encouraged to track the changes in their stress levels over time and to note in the accompanying app external life events and activity patterns (relating to work, sleep and socialising) that may explain the changes in galvanic skin response that the device measures. The Moodmetric app is described as a 'stress management tool' that can be integrated with the user's diary and notes records. Here, again, we see indirect acknowledgement that it is not possible to understand physiological stress without also tracking one's emotional and practical life. One needs to develop answers to questions like: what did I do on those days when my skin response was atypical? Does arriving home from work correlate with higher or lower skin temperatures? How does my meditation class affect my skin temperature data? The use of the word 'mood' to describe the ring is notable here: like the popular 1970s' novelties of the same name, the changing colours of the ring are meant to indicate something much more than skin temperature. Skin temperature is, in other words, not sufficient even in the manufacturer's discourse to understand one's stress or mood.

The need to document relevant life events and to correlate them with biosensing data resonates with many of the fertility sensors discussed in Chapter 1. In both cases, correlation work takes place on biodigital platforms and can involve focusing on oneself (the $n = 1$) and/or comparison with others (those constituting the imagined 'n = all').[2] When using the Temperature Egg, for example, users manually enter data about pain, sexual intercourse and bleeding on the device itself, or via the associated app. This data then becomes part of a package sent to 'experts' to analyse (that is, to feed into their algorithm-building process). Similarly, in apps such as Clue or Glow, users are encouraged to enter a diverse set of data about sexual energy or drive, sexual encounters, mood, and physical changes. The need for additional documentation in the cases of both stress and fertility monitoring place burdens on users, and tends to undermine manufacturers' claims that self-tracking is easy or simple. Small-scale qualitative studies of stress biosensing have found that some participants experience the process as burdensome and, indeed, stress-inducing (Tucker and Goodings, 2015; Pantzar and Ruckenstein, 2017). Devices may well facilitate the collection of some forms of data (basal body temperature or skin conductivity), and associated computer interfaces may present correlative graphs of information collected (for example, number of steps and hours of REM [Rapid Eye Movement] sleep), but there are thousands of other measures that they cannot yet take: how much sex you have[3]; what your

---

[2] Such comparisons are discussed in more detail in Chapter 4.

[3] Some men do apparently use accelerometers on their wrist-worn devices to measure thrust frequency and heart rate during sexual intercourse

subjective mood is; and whether you are menstruating and how painful an experience that is.

Making sense of biosensing data, then, requires 'older' forms of data collection and storage: genealogical histories, diaries, note-taking and self-awareness. As both Wilkinson and Kragh-Furbo found in their ethnographic studies (of fertility monitoring and direct-to-consumer genetic testing, respectively), it also frequently involves the ancient art of conversation and dialogue, written or spoken. Biosensing data rarely, if ever, 'speaks for itself'. It has to be platformised, that is, interpreted, analysed and titrated with other data, lived experience and existing knowledges.

One device – the Bellabeat Leaf Urban – promises to inform users of their 'stress preparedness' each day by accumulating an individual's biosensing and hand-entered data:

> In essence, it takes all the tracking we've mentioned and pulls it together to give you a score – as an in-app visualisation – showing how ready you are to deal with stress that day. And how that compares to yesterday. That's based on how well rested you are, whether you've meditated or exercised and what point in your menstrual cycle you're at. (Charara, 2016)

Like other biosensing devices and apps, the Bellabeat Leaf Urban is also oriented towards teaching users to directly influence their bodies in order to reduce stress, in this case, via breathing coaching. Other devices focus more directly on the brain: 'Muse', for example, involves a tightly-worn headband containing seven EEG (electroencephalogram) sensors that

---

(Lupton, 2015), while in 2014, a penis-worn, wireless prototype device was advertised that could count thrusts and calories burned, and provides a set of flashing LED lights to aid thrust rhythm (see Levy, 2015).

register electrical neurological activity. Users work though guided meditation sessions, with the device providing audio feedback about how well they are managing to control their neurological activity (see Figure 2.2). Described in an online review as 'meditation for geeks', this device is an excellent example of the ways in which contemporary stress biosensing relies both on biofeedback science and on Eastern traditions of meditation and mindfulness (Charara, 2015).

Figure 2.2: 'Muse'

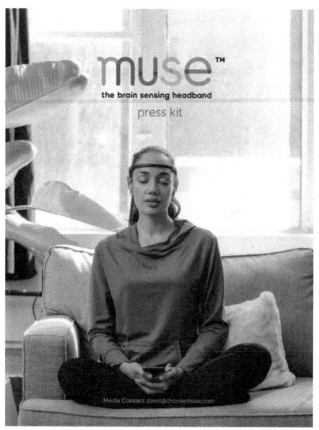

Source: Copyright of Muse (www.choosemuse.com); Caddy (2018)

Stress surveillance?

The ability to record physiological shifts over time is key to contemporary biosensing. One could argue that it is fundamental – the reason that studying an 'n = 1' makes any sense at all. As Dawn Nafus (2016a: xix) puts it, 'Sensors lay tracks in time'. Measuring stress through galvanic skin response or heart-rate variability allows individuals to track their 'levels' in real time and to make associations between life events (stressors) and physiological signs. (As Pantzar and Ruckenstein [2017: 5; see also Pantzar et al, 2017] found, such associations, or lack thereof, can be surprising: one participant in their study of heart-rate variability monitoring found that intense shouting fights with her husband elicited no signs of stress.) Of course, the apps could also help others to make such connections. The Moodmetric website also offers a service to companies wishing to track 'executive stress' through two to eight weeks of measurement 'complemented with assisting services', whatever those might be (Meditation classes? Redundancy planning?) (see: www.moodmetric.com/products/).[4] Other consumer-oriented discourses similarly argue that employers could use stress data to know when an employee is best able to work. A 2015 article in the *Financial Review* (2015), for example, entitled 'Why your boss wants you to wear biosensing devices', claimed:

[S]cience is starting to show that some hormones – including naturally produced steroids and testosterone – increase confidence and make us take more risks. Meanwhile stress hormones like cortisol produce the opposite effect.

---

[4] In her trenchant popular critique of the 'multi-billion pound [stress] industry' and, indeed, of the concept of 'stress' itself, Angela Patmore (2006: 206) quotes a 'Stressdots' manufacturer who claims that the dots

Wearable technology – be it heart-rate monitors or skin response sensors – can give this underlying influence more visibility, says Coates. "You need to figure out whether you should be trading or whether you should go home. If you are trading, should you double up your position because you're in the zone?"

This article suggests that employers in the financial industry, in motor racing and in the military are already using stress biosensing to determine who should be doing what work. In online research, we did find that stress biosensing systems – measuring heart rate, galvanic skin response and/or EEG patterns – are, indeed, recommended for use in military contexts to assess the capacity of soldiers to cope with combat and other situations (Hoyt et al, 2002; Arcana and Indira, 2013; Montgomery and Anderson, 2016; Ciorap, 2017). These systems are embedded in uniforms and worn devices, and work alongside GPS tracking devices and temperature monitors to provide continuous information about each soldier, supposedly comparing data to each individual's typical state (Ciorap, 2017).

Could such devices ethically be used by parents to assess children's stress? As mentioned in Box 2.1, adoptive parents and foster carers in the UK, the US and elsewhere are encouraged to come to connect their children's behaviours and feelings not only to early life (including in utero) experiences of suffering and loss, but also to physiological and neurological states and patterns arising from these experiences. Levels of stress hormones are key here: cortisol flows are, as mentioned earlier, thought to be disrupted by early life trauma and to establish atypical patterns that endure into adulthood. For parents and carers, then, as Winnicottian therapist Christine Bradley (2017:78) writes in

---

are used by companies to inform redundancy decisions. Nissenbaum and Patterson (2016) provide helpful analysis of employers' interests in employees' biosensing data in the US.

her 2017 book *Revealing the inner world of traumatised children and young people*, for example: 'Understanding about cortisol is useful. The chemical cortisol is released in the brain during stress, its purpose along with adrenaline is to activate preparedness for flight or fight when in danger. In excess, however, due to ongoing stress it begins to have a toxic effect.' Importantly, Bradley (2017: 78–9) (and others producing this discourse) figure cortisol levels as something that can be altered through caring interactions, with therapists and/or parents and carers:

> Emotional stressful factors causing anxiety, depression and insomnia have an effect on hormones in the body and brain, but this does not have to be a permanent state of affairs. Cortisol levels can be influenced by reparative care, and the effects of chronic stress can be alleviated.

Interestingly, at least as far as we are aware, none of these therapists currently recommend biosensing as a way to understand a child's stress levels. Instead, they suggest that physiological signs of stress are read in the face and embodiment of the child and in the carer's own bodily sensations (see, for example, Hughes and Baylin, 2012). This advice builds on the already-honed skills of facial reading that most parents and carers develop, but tends to require a lot of learning about one's own physiological stress reactions. Some researchers, in contrast, suggest that measuring cortisol in saliva might help foster carers understand their charges. In a 2017 review of relevant research literature, for example, Van Andel et al (2014: 10) suggest that 'diurnal cortisol with a wake up and a bedtime measurement may be a relevant tool to evaluate stress in young foster children' who are too young to articulate their feelings clearly (or, indeed, who are habituated to feeling stressed and so are less able to recognise or report it). Such measurements, the authors suggest, might also be used to indicate the value of foster carers' interventions to help reduce stress.

Rather more directly than devices such as Fitbits or Moodmetric rings, or over-the-counter cortisol tests, this research enters into the difficult territory of gaps between physiological stress and 'felt stress', encountering the complex fault lines between what is 'normal' (either statistically or in terms of health) and what is 'normalised'. Van Andel et al (2014) describe children as unable to know their own stress, and foster carers as struggling to assess outward signs of distress. Other studies have confirmed that measurements of physiological stress (as measured, for example, in saliva cortisol levels) often do not correlate well with felt stress. In a review of studies looking at 'the associations between physiological and psychological responses' to stressors, for example, Campbell and Ehlert (2012: 1111) find only a 25 per cent correlation. This could be because individuals who are exposed to long-term stressors and/or who experience early life trauma may become highly accustomed to the physiological experience of stress, so that they experience it as 'normal'. A more critical take could be that this differential indicates that 'stress' is a meaningless concept (for a version of this argument, see Patmore, 2006). In any case, it is important to consider the possible tensions of an articulation of stress that prioritises physiological signs over lived experience. While individuals might sometimes experience counter-intuitive physiological measurements as interesting, even helpful (as did some of Pantzar and Ruckenstein's [2017] participants), there are risks that cortisol levels or skin conductivity could be used to judge fostering practices as inadequate, for example, despite a child presenting as, or being felt by carers to be, non-stressed. It seems to us that it remains hugely important to critically triangulate any stress biosensing data and to view such data as always–already social (rather than simply factual).

What is peculiar to stress monitoring, when compared to more widespread biosensing practices such as step counting or ovulation monitoring, is that the measuring may directly (that is, physiologically) affect what is being measured. Indeed, it is meant to do so: stress monitoring is intended to reduce distress and ideally to improve people's lived experience. However, as 'white coat syndrome' famously does for blood pressure (when an individual's blood pressure rises when measured by a doctor), might simply measuring one's stress sometimes increase it? The wager of scientists and manufacturers of stress apps, tests and biosensors is that measuring is a physiologically neutral practice – that, like step counters or ovulation monitors, biosensing simply measures and documents something that is already there. Stress, however, is a multifaceted and complex phenomenon that is, by its nature, already psychosocial. There can be no neutral measuring here (see also Tucker and Goodings, 2015). Developers of these platforms also assume that users will act appropriately when warned that their stress levels are high – that they will act, in other words, to reduce their stress. Studies of other forms of biosensing, however, such as the use of activity monitors for weight loss, show the opposite. Reports in major medical journals such as the *British Medical Journal* and *Journal of the American Medical Association* (*JAMA*), for example, have shown that wearing a device (even when cash incentives are also offered) does not change exercise or eating behaviours, and that people who monitor their food intake and exercise through other means are more likely to lose weight than those using biosensors and apps (Wise, 2016). Although some participants in Pantzar and Ruckenstein's (2017) study of heart-rate variability said that they were going to try to change their behaviour to reduce their stress (for example, avoiding arguing with their partner late at night), others highlighted that the events that seemed to trigger stress responses felt outside their control (for example, sleeping badly after an acrimonious divorce).

The collective politics of stress

Although stress testing and monitoring could be used to make consequential judgements about others (Are employees coping with their work? Are foster carers looking after children properly?), all of the figurations of stress monitoring discussed to this point have focused on individuals and/or interpersonal relationships (such as parent–child or fostering relationships). However, does stress biosensing inevitably lead us in the individualising direction?

While researching this chapter, one of us travelled to the US and was introduced to a research group at the University of Illinois who are using stress biosensing (specifically heart-rate variation monitoring) to do something rather different. In this study, Ruby Mendenhall, Christy Lleras and colleagues are gathering data on African-American mothers' experiences of stress relating to gun violence in inner-city Chicago. As well as monitoring heart rate and physical movement through wearable biosensors, they are collecting women's felt experiences through written and visual diaries, and collating data on gun crime via environmental sensors, cameras and police data. In informal discussions, Mendenhall and Lleras stated that women involved in the project had welcomed both the physiological data on elevated heart rate and the environmental and police data on gunshots as confirmation of their felt experience of fear and anxiety around crime events. Importantly, however, the central aim of the project is to collect data in order, through visualisation and public exhibition, to render the experience of gun-related violence more collective and, in that way, more amenable to policy and social change. Mendenhall et al (2018) write:

> Our final product will be the development of an affective diary platform that will be used to document how violence affects public life and public health in the 'hidden America'. The affective diaries will include unique visualizations of the complex data and will be used as a tool to empower African American mothers to communicate how exposure to community violence affects their collective health and

organize around changes in health policy and public policy more broadly.

Ultimately, the value of this kind of work will depend on how the data is transformed through the collection, comparison and contrasting enabled by platforms. Little will be gained if differences between forms of data remain unexplored, or if their divergent histories of value are ignored: women's written testimony has a very different cultural and scientific valence compared to heart-rate calculations or police crime data. Critical triangulation should open up ontological and epistemological questions about the object of study, in this case, about the nature of stress, the physiology of heart rate and the social capacity of humans to testify to their own experience in written or spoken form (see also Convery et al, 2008). It must also resist demanding that particular people or groups take care of their physiology without necessary social change.

Nikolas Rose and Joelle Abi-Rached (2013: 231) describe a similar study by Meyer-Lindenberg et al on urbanicity, stress and mental disorder. Criticising the neuroscientists' claims to 'a new empirical approach for integrating social sciences, neurosciences and public policy to respond to the major health challenge of urbanization' (Lederbogen et al, 2011: 500), they argue that such research will only have value if it can engage in genuinely open conversation with critical social science and learn from:

> a century of empirical research and conceptualization in sociology, social history, and cultural geography on these issues, on the ways in which they play out in the mental lives of the inhabitants of these environments, and on the policy difficulties that are entailed in transforming the experiences and consequences of contemporary forms of urban life. (Rose and Abi-Rached, 2013: 232)

We are in agreement with Rose and Abi-Rached on this point.

Biosensing stress, in this kind of collaborative, connecting work, has the potential to help researchers and citizens to think about the ways in which external worlds, internal physiological processes and lived experience are enmeshed or imbricated. While those living in dangerous parts of cities, of course, already know that that is a stressful experience, biosensing can articulate some of their physiological reactions to specific stressors such as gunshots. Similarly, while politicians and policymakers should already recognise the difficulties associated with living in such conditions, they may be more likely to act if 'hard evidence' of the physical correlates of such experiences is gathered via sensors. Here, then, biosensing becomes a platform for collective politics – both to affirm shared experience (through the collection and comparison of individuals' data) and to lobby for change.[5] In such studies, stress biosensing moves further away from step counting or even ovulation monitoring and becomes more like direct-to-consumer genetic testing, where the pooling and sharing of data are what render any particular individual's data meaningful (see Chapter 3). This more politicised use of biosensing data also has strong potential links to forms of environmental sensing used by community activists to document water, air or food pollution (see, for example, work in Japan post-Fukushima [Kimura and Inose, forthcoming] and on water quality in Indonesia [Böhlen, 2016]).

This version of biosensing may open up understandings of 'the social' to include forms of human connection other than interpersonal or familial settings. Here, importantly, communities, suburbs and other forms of spatial groupings can 'count'. What is less positive, on the other hand, is that such uses run the risk of reducing stress to an accumulation of external stressors, overlooking or underplaying the role of personal

---

[5]   For studies of the ways in which health activists use collected stories to influence both policy and scientific research, see Rabeharisoa, Moreira and Akrich (2014).

histories and physiologies in the experience of stress. There is much work to be done, we suggest, in learning how to bridge between collective and individual experiences in this field.

Conclusions

Stress biosensing as currently marketed clearly articulates a cultural logic that assumes that knowing about one's internal bodily states is healthy and that measuring stress will have no negative effects. From the literature on stress and Mackenzie and Roberts's (2017) autoethnographic study of adoptive parenting, however, we learn that stress involves complex, relational and situated processes. In contemporary adoption training, parents are taught how to recognise signs of distress in children with histories of early life trauma: these may include changes in movement, eye focus and tone of voice, but are also felt in the bodies of parents (for example, one's own heart rate may increase). Parents are trained to use their own bodies to regulate their child's stress response: to alter their own breathing; to stroke their own skin; and to modulate their voices. Such training articulates (di)stress in relational and embodied ways, combining mental, social and physical actions in sometimes surprising ways (Mackenzie and Roberts, 2017). It would be hard to imagine a biosensing system that could function in such a nuanced way. This is not to argue, to be clear, that stress biosensing is an inevitably useless endeavour. As discussed earlier, we can imagine times and places in which particular measurements might help to articulate bodies in politically helpful or health-oriented exploratory ways. Biosensing stress might, for example, help parents to understand (and explain to others) the ways in which current (di)stress relates to early abuse or neglect, and thus to contest mainstream understandings of their children's 'behavioural difficulties' in health and educational settings.

In the conclusion to her edited book on biosensing, Nafus (2016a: 228) writes:

> It's clear that biosensors do not make anyone's life "simpler,"
> contrary to the claims of product manufacturers. Rather,
> a biosensor-rich world requires a much more complex
> notion of where a person's body begins and ends.

The same could, arguably, be said for stress: understanding stress
requires a much more complex notion of where a person's body
begins and ends. We disagree with Looker and Gregson's claim
(with which we started this chapter) that 'stress' is just something
within you; instead, we suggest that stress problematises any
clear distinction between inside and outside, or between
'self' and 'other'. Stress also problematises conventional ideas
of the individualised, linear 'life course': people who have
endured severe early life stress experience recurring embodied
difficulties – forms of bodily memory – that are also felt by
others living with or caring for them. As with other hormonal
processes, the physiological processes articulating stress are, in
our view, biopsychosocial (Roberts, 2007, 2015). Biosensing
stress, then, will be at its most useful when it becomes a way of
articulating this complexity rather than a tool to shut it down.
Used in this way, attempts to biosense the 'indicators' of stress
may help laypeople, scientists and clinicians to develop more
complex understandings of the imbrications of human biology
and lived, situated experience, and thus to develop more
sustaining conceptions of the (healthy) life course.

3

Platform Biosensing and Post-Genomic Relatedness

The biosensing practice concerning us in this chapter bears different names: DNA genotyping, genetic tests or personal genomics. But it targets a single macro-molecule shared by all living things, DNA. DNA genotyping begins with a tissue sample, usually taken from saliva.[1] Where it ends is difficult to say. Since 2007, DNA genotyping has been available 'direct' to 'consumers'. In this context, 'direct' means without recourse to a medical clinic or medical pathology services. The tests, sometimes called 'direct-to-consumer' (DTC) genetic tests, are direct in the sense that people submit their saliva and payment from home rather than at a doctor's clinic or medical facility, and results come back to them rather than to a physician. In many respects, the tests are indirect. They depend on social network platforms, they leverage publicly funded scientific research and they struggle to comprehend and capitalise on test results whose

---

[1] Since DNA is the most extensively discussed biomolecule barring none, we say nothing much about it here. We note, however, that biological techniques for working with DNA have displayed a marked tendency to 'double down' on DNA for the last three to four decades. That is, each time DNA is sequenced or otherwise manipulated, and some knowledge or understanding derives from that, the investment in sequencing or otherwise manipulating it seems to double, as if that first glimpse of worth lures scientists to pursue it twice or ten times as far. In the past five decades, this has led to a proliferation of devices, techniques, projects, forms of expertise, scientific knowledge infrastructures, products, institutions, services and performances associated with DNA.

significance snakes around plural variations of patterns of DNA. They are steeped in practices and patterns of biomedical and Internet platformisation that precede and expand beyond them. The genotyping platforms, with their devices – for example, DNA chips or microarrays – and scientific entourage (genome-wide association studies [GWAS], DNA genotyping data and literature databases, and so on) – build on wider transformations in biology, life sciences and biomedicine. They are rooted in the exigencies of institutional health care, online platforms and the changing relations of states to their citizens.[2] DNA genotyping platforms – our preferred term for the biosensing dimension of DTC genetic tests – display all the messy entanglements of selfhood, relatedness, regulation, health, science, technology, platform capitalism and collective sense-making visible in biosensing more widely.

This chapter describes some key aspects of the burgeoning of DNA biosensing, bringing into focus its attachment to Internet platforms, ambivalence towards clinical expertise, speculation on future scientific knowledge and embrace of 'data citizenship'. In terms of biosensing practices and the life course, DNA genotyping ostensibly concerns the problem of future risks or susceptibilities (for example, of Alzheimer's disease or macular degeneration), some or many of which endure beyond the course of an individual life. However, as we will suggest, DNA biosensing stretches above and beyond risk calculations or predictions of individual health outcomes. The biosensing of DNA genotyping promises future understanding and, like so

---

[2] The citizens' panel we conducted on DTC genetic testing frequently raised questions of who profits from DNA testing and who does not. Participants consistently voiced their trust in clinical expertise and publicly funded health-care providers. Their concerns are writ large in regulatory controversies associated with 23andMe and, to a less extent, other DNA testing services in recent years (2013–18). In certain ways, the expert panels of medical practitioners, public health advocates and civil society commentators affirmed the citizens' concerns around profit.

much biosensing, future devices. Although genotyping fits the definition of biosensing that we started from ('understanding changes in body state' [see Introduction]), DNA biosensors do not, as yet, exist as wearable or implantable devices. Like nanotechnology biosensors, DNA biosensors exist as a promise. The Wikipedia article on biosensors, for instance, states: 'in the future, DNA will find use as a versatile material from which scientists can craft biosensors. DNA biosensors can theoretically be used for medical diagnostics, forensic science, agriculture, or even environmental clean-up efforts. No external monitoring is needed for DNA-based sensing devices' (Wikipedia, 2017).[3] 'Will find use' are the key words. As we will see, DNA-derived data is already important in some forms of biosensing associated with specific health conditions, especially so-called 'functional disorders' such as chronic fatigue syndrome. But because DNA registers so many changes and variations in body state, DNA data percolates through biosensing practice more broadly, sometimes forming the substrate or platform on which other forms of biosensing stand. The Infinome Project (Infinome, 2018) endeavours, for instance, to bring together DTC genetic data with exercising tracking data to manage obesity. The connotation of the name 'Infinome' is typical of DNA biosensing: expansion is planned.

By virtue of its platformised materiality (the fact that DNA sequencing powers up on an assemblage of sequencers and databases [Stevens, 2011] and poetics [Roof, 2007]), DNA is a potent indicator of body state. As a biomolecule, it spans an extraordinary range of body and environment relations, including many forms of variation and exchange such as sexual reproduction and heredity. In 20th-century biology, DNA

---

[3]   Recent scientific publications suggest that the Wikipedia article on biosensors needs updating. Many articles on DNA biosensors appear in recent scientific literature (Khan et al, 2016), although none have resulted in commercially available products.

figured centrally in the redefinition of life as a signal processing system. Contemporary DNA biosensing practices inhabit a wider ecology of scientific work that we might term 'post-genomic'. They follow in the wake of the completion of the sequencing of the human genome in 2001 (Richardson and Stevens, 2015), and they betray signs of an unevenly distributed awareness that genomes – the full complement of DNA of an organism – and genes do not so much control or programme biological processes as register their sensitivity to cross-hybridisation, mutations, relationality and variation. The many *-omes* proliferating in the wake of genomes – proteome, metabolome, interactome, microbiome and, more recently, exposome – are one sign of this expanding awareness of DNA's relatedness.

Perhaps the defining feature of DNA biosensing practices is the mobility of DNA sequence and other genomic data. It has spilled out of laboratory and clinical records. The mobility of DNA data affects its significance in biosensing practice. In 2018, as we write, it has become easy to move DNA-related data between platforms, analytical tools and visualisations. Some of the authors have downloaded, uploaded, shared and interpreted their own genotype data with little technical effort. A 650,000-line plain-text file on a hard drive can contain genotype data for an individual. After several decades of DNA sequencing, the growth of a specialised sub-discipline of computer science and biology largely focused on sequence data (bioinformatics), and some very large global consortia projects focused on genomes, the mundane details of file formats, the specifications of scientific instruments and biosensors such as microarrays, and the statistical steps needed to identify significant correlations and patterns in sequence data have stabilised and even become standardised. This allows DNA data to circulate well beyond the scientific databases and knowledge infrastructures it initially inhabited.

The platformisation of genotyping – the specification of the genetic variations that differentiate an individual from a population – expands the scope of the reinterpretation or contestation of biological differences. Platforms afford comparison of individual genomes. Like many platform interactions, the comparisons lend weight to variations and differences. Such variations and differences can be used to individualise disease. They foster the emergence of the idea of personalising medicine (Tutton, 2016). Not only does genomics afford the individualisation of disease, it also encourages a variational understanding of disease as the outcome of a set of interactions specific to a unique life history. Researchers sometimes speak of unique disease rather than illnesses defined by population-based measures (for instance, of blood pressure or heart rate).

It is feasible that elementary forms of clinical citizenship are altered via DNA genotyping platforms. The significance of measures or imputations of discrete risks is changing. Genetic risks for specific disease, in their association with the harm, suffering, damage, severity, downsides and costs of care, stand at the centre of much clinical experience, expertise and practice. Risks in the form of susceptibilities to inherited diseases have been the primary focus of clinical genetics and public health policies for at least a century (Keller, 2001, 2005). Biopolitical governmentality is the ensemble of medical and health practices, discourses and institutions that has made these risks one of its primary problems. In turn, patients, citizens and consumers actively engage with genetic risks, remaking their own lives in the process. As Nikolas Rose (2007: 107) writes:

> genetics takes its salience within a political and ethical field in which individuals are increasingly obligated to formulate life strategies, to seek to maximize their life chance, to take actions or refrain from actions in order to increase the quality of their lives, and to act prudently in relation to themselves and others.

Genetic risk relates to future outcomes and expectations calculated for a particular disease or condition with reference to the norms of a population. Quantifications of risk using probabilities and valuations of the severity of outcomes seek to manage uncertainty through calculations whose efficacy and reliability derive from clinical trials and studies of patients. The risk calculations for specific diseases or conditions, including those of population-wide public health campaigns, remain narrowly focused in comparison to the gamut of variations entertained in DNA biosensing. It is striking that risk-related information from DNA genetic tests has often been less interesting to their recipients. As Martin Richards (2010: 1) writes, risks are often 'skeptically interpreted through a frame of knowledge of family disease histories'. This scepticism is well founded. Even after more than a decade of intense research efforts, genotyped predictions of genetic risk remain notoriously unreliable (for instance, different DNA testing services supply divergent risk estimates for conditions like Alzheimer's disease [Hercher, 2018]).[4]

If DNA biosensing expands and generalises genetic risk calculations into a broad-spectrum profiling of propensities and susceptibilities, varying between people and over time, we would expect DNA biosensing to affect experiences of what it is to be alive or to be living. DNA genotyping platforms lie in the fault zone between biology and medicine. They emerge in the middle of the unstable relation between life as form and life as experience of health and illness. Taking stock of the platforms and configurations devised to sense and understand DNA data, and attending to slippages as DNA data traverses spaces between clinics and various database and social media platforms, is one

---

[4] We might also point to the fact that many DNA tests offer information about ancestry alongside health.

way in which we might get a sense of how this change in experience of biological vitality occurs.[5]

Understanding the tests

What in DNA genotyping diverges from the biopolitical governmentality of risk, an institutional–individual engagement that not only draws people into treatments, but also to novel diets and foods, exercise programmes, and alternative therapies? Does DNA genotyping react to risk along the lines that many social science health researchers have explored in the context of genetic disease, addiction, chronic disease or mental ill health? On good statistical grounds and to skirt around the government regulation of medical testing devices, DNA testing platforms such as 23andMe have tended to avoid making claims to calculate individual health risks: 'The tests are not intended to diagnose a disease, or tell you anything about your risk for developing a disease in the future' (23andMe, 2018a).

In practice, much of the information they provide to their customers is risk-oriented. They provide information about increased risks of diseases such as Alzheimer's and Parkinson's, but they do not always prominently say that genetic risk is thought to account for a small portion of the overall risk. 23andMe invites people to see themselves through the instrument of DNA testing, and stages the DNA genotyping as a version of self – 'Welcome to You' is printed across the 23andMe testkit box – but the version of self in play here is not the medical subject or the citizen-patient of biopolitics. Who is welcomed here?

---

[5]   There is a slender possibility too that DNA biosensing is a pragmatic thought style attuned to new relationships between life and human sciences. As Nikolas Rose (2013: 5) writes, 'thought styles are emerging in many areas of contemporary biology that offer the opportunity for a new relationship between the human sciences and the life sciences'.

A large and growing body of social research has analysed DTC genetic tests from their inception, and this literature continues to grow (Saukko, 2009; Bloss et al, 2010; Richards, 2010; Hauskeller, 2011; Harris et al, 2016). The research frequently discusses 23andMe, a company that has sold genetic testing as a service over the Internet since 2007. The tests are also provided by firms such as FamilyTreeDNA, Ancestry.com, Genos, MyHeritage and LivingDNA.[6] Some of these services report the DNA genotyping tests results, but many also offer analysis, interpretation and further information on genealogy, ethnicity and kinship. More specialised analysis platforms such as DNA. land, codegen, openSNP, Genes for Good and Promethease provide more specialised analysis and interpretation. The two key issues addressed in social research and wider debates concerning 23andMe and similar companies, such as the now-defunct deCodeMe and Navigenics, or newer entrants such ubiome, have been the relation between DTC genetic tests and medical expertise, and the commercial uses of the data. Problems of regulation and knowledge, of ethics and epistemology, have been at the forefront of the discussions.

In our research, we approach DNA genotyping from the standpoint of biosensing. Practically, we focus on how data produced by biosensors is understood. We ask: what happens to the data after it leaves the biosensor? Where does it go? How is it transformed? Where is it merged or stacked up with other data? We observe that since their appearance more than a decade ago, the variety of platforms and the network of associated databases and analytical tools has greatly increased. DNA genotyping presents a much more complex ecology of biosensing than any image of a diagnostic test conveys. Like many other contemporary biosensings, the trajectory of the data from biosensor to understanding is a convoluted one,

---

[6]   A listing of health and ancestry testing services at dnatestingchoice.com
     shows around 200 different services.

passing through analytical pipelines that often involve automated machine learning or other forms of prediction or imputation. In work that forms a backdrop for this chapter, we have explored the transformations in data analysis associated with machine learning (Mackenzie, 2017), the emergence of global scientific knowledge infrastructures for DNA sequence data (Stevens, 2011) and the development of large-scale platform deployments for prediction (Mackenzie, 2018), and via a citizen's panel, we have explored public concerns about the ownership of DNA genotyping data. More specifically, we draw on case studies carried about by Mette Kragh-Furbo as part of her PhD work on how DNA genotyping data circulates beyond the edges of the platforms on which it was produced (see Box 3.1). We take a particular interest in some cases where the so-called 'raw data' (shown in the sample) moves and in moving changes. These cases include some of the authors' own DNA genotyping data; this chapter, like others in this book, has an autoethnographic element.

The complexity of genotyping as biosensing is partly attributable to the biosensor in question: the microarray. Microarrays are sometimes called 'lab on a chip'. 23andMe uses 'a custom Illumina HumanOmniExpress-24 format chip' (23andMe, 2018f). The microarray is a matchbox-sized spotted plate. The plate typically contains around 700,000 spots or points at which DNA sequences have been fixed in known locations. In a microarray system, which is a biomedical platform in Paul Keating and Alberto Cambrosio's (2003) sense of the term, prepared biological samples – the saliva submitted to 23andMe travels in a plastic tube via FedEx – flow over the plate. Fragments of DNA in the sample bond or 'hybridise' to varying degrees with spots on the plate. A digital imaging system sensitive to the fluorescence of the bonded spots measures the intensity of the binding at each spot. Each location on the microarray chip, with its selected and designed DNA sequence, effectively constitutes a test. So, in the data sample shown in Table 3.1, the rsid column

Table 3.1: Sample of genotyping data on chromosome 1 from a
23andMe data download

Rsid	Chrom	Position	Genotype
rs548049170	1	69869	TT
rs13328684	1	74792	–
rs9283150	1	565508	AA
i713426	1	726912	–
rs116587930	1	727841	GG
rs3131972	1	752721	AG

lists single nucleotide polymorphism (SNP) IDs that flag known
locations in the three billion or so elements in the genome. The
array of tests on a microarray permits in the order of a million
tests to be made on a given sample. Although some biosensors
produce periodic or even streams of measurements over time,
the microarray as a biosensor makes hundreds of thousands
of readings all at one point in time. What it lacks in temporal
continuity, it replaces with parallelism.

The array of 700,000 tests, each of which potentially relates
to a distinct risk, pathology or physiological trait, seems to
intensify or even hyperbolically multiply risks. With that
many tests on a single DNA sample, do we witness a massive
expansion of risk awareness or risk-oriented knowledges?
Is DNA biosensing expanding risk? Yes and no. Perhaps for
the first time in the history of medicine, people can access
a broad spectrum of risk-related information about many
different health-related matters; in this respect, DTC genetic
testing is a foretaste of the much more heavily instrumented
development of clinical genomic or precision medicine in
which medical diagnosis and treatment will routinely begin
with full sequencing of the genome of individual patients. At
the same time, the multiplication of tests in DNA biosensing
diffuses into a very indeterminate and future-oriented approach
to health in which propensities and susceptibilities to disease
stand side by side with indications of metabolic, nervous,

biomechanical or digestive specificities. The indeterminacy and breadth of the genotyping tests is such that clinicians typically find them of little use. Even clinical geneticists testing for genetic diseases, such as Huntington's, which are relatively rare and are usually well known to people through family history, or for more common forms of heart disease, do not typically use microarray genotyping.

From the perspective of biosensing practices, the diffuse, broad spectrum of tests performed in DNA genotyping is not necessarily a problem. On the contrary, the indeterminacies may generate interesting practices in the wild, beyond the regulated forms of clinical expertise. As devices, microarrays, perhaps more than some of the other biosensors that we have been discussing, depend on and engage with scientific knowledges. Those knowledges configure the microarrays themselves. The many DNA fragments on the microarray are chosen because they represent SNPs. An SNP is a single change in the G,C, A or T nucleotides in a given DNA sequence (US National Library of Medicine, 2018). The set of SNPs represented on the microarray not only profiles an individual genotype, but also snapshots a state of scientific knowledge at a point in time. It distils in miniature thousands of scientific studies. Microarrays change as new scientific literature and data sets appear, and genotyping results are also subject to ongoing revision. From time to time, 23andMe, for instance, supplies new results or reports to its customers.

SNPs, of which there are millions in a human genome, occur in population-specific patterns. Contemporary genomic science adheres to the hypothesis that the distribution of these patterns can be used to genotype an individual in relation to a population. DNA genotyping using microarrays is predicated on the idea that the distribution of SNPs offers a profile of how an individual differs from a population in relation to ancestry, in relation to susceptibility to environmental factors and in relation to inherited disease. History, environment and health are signalled by SNPs in different ways: sometimes because the SNP is a signpost marking population differences (blue eyes, cleft chin, hair on the back); sometimes because the SNP is part of a gene whose biological function may contribute to disease (late-onset Parkinson's, sickle cell anaemia) or relations to the environment (metabolises caffeine and other similar toxins slowly); and most often because the patterns of association between a number of SNPs correlates to a certain degree with physiological traits, pathologies or other attributes. Although each spot on the microarray tests for the presence of a single SNP in the biological sample, the pattern of tests for SNPs, those whose marker status may relate to ancestry, environment or inherited disease, suggests the possibility of many different combinations of tests, combinations that may crisscross lineages of populations, environmental conditions and familial heredity. These combinatorial possibilities create a risk terrain whose topography can no longer be viewed solely in terms of isolated peaks of risk. It invites open-ended exploration of associations.

We get some sense of the remarkably dense interweaving of a device with fields of science in the diagram of GWAS (see Figure 3.1). In this diagram, the 23 chromosomes of the human genome are islands populated by scientific studies. Each chromosome has many SNPs. Each grey scaled dot represents a scientific study that has analysed some pattern of association between the SNPs and a physiological trait or state of interest to researchers. Exploring how the biological and medical sciences have oriented themselves to this combinatorial expansion of tests and multi-factor risk calculation would take us far afield. We simply note that tests selected for inclusion on the biosensor – the spots on the array – depend on the prior art of scientific studies that have identified associations between SNPs in particular populations, diseases and other body states.

At least 10,000 GWAS have taken place since 2000. These GWAS and their affiliated publications erect the scaffolding on which both the biosensor as a platform and the platformisation

Figure 3.1: Diagram of genome-wide association studies

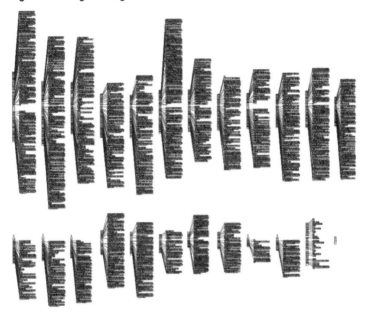

Source: Copyright of EMBL-EBI 2017; Buniello et al (2019)

of genotyping as a service stands.[7] The GWAS constitute a shape-shifting mass of scientific knowledge. On the one hand, they catalogue a variety of associations between DNA genotypes and common conditions. Table 3.2 shows a count of GWAS studies focused on different human and disease traits. Close to 1,000 GWAS concern obesity, 800 concern height, 700 concern immunity, 350 concern diabetes and so forth. Cholesterol or breast cancer are hardly surprising targets of study. On the other hand, browsing the GWAS catalogue (such as: www.ebi.ac.uk/gwas/search/traits) quickly shows that the traits investigated by GWAS fan out across educational

---

[7] A useful account of the development of GWAS in the context of personalised medicine can be found in Tutton (2016).

Table 3.2: Top ten traits in GWAS according to ebicat38

Trait	Number of GWAS
Obesity-related traits	957
Height	822
IgG glycosylation	699
Type 2 diabetes	340
Rheumatoid arthritis	294
Crohn's disease	249
Schizophrenia	248
Blood metabolite levels	245
HDL cholesterol	222
Breast cancer	199

attainment, loneliness, cluster headaches, political preferences and coffee consumption, through to coughing types and head circumference. Especially in the area of behavioural genetics, many GWAS can claim only tenuous credibility (Panofsky, 2015). The traits they aim to investigate using patterns of statistically significant co-occurrence of SNPs sometimes lack coherence. Political preference or entrepreneurship is hardly a distinct phenotypical attribute like eye colour. GWAS combine the statistical credibility of large cohort studies, high-throughput laboratory automation and an extensively cross-linked knowledge infrastructure (for an account of this, see Kragh-Furbo et al, 2016). They sometimes foray into areas of human 'behaviour' that even the most aggressive biomedicalising ambitions have not ventured to treat clinically.

Share and compare?

GWAS studies lend a vital buoyancy to DNA-based biosensing. When a 23andMe customer finds that they have, say, 91 reports waiting for them in their login member area, reports that provide individual risk estimates ranging across many of the traits that we have just glimpsed in passing, they step into a current of biosensing flowing out of a global techno-assemblage. The reports bob around in a wide genomic sea of studies. Customers' sense of agency is both excited and overwhelmed in the face of the reports. The multiplication of studies, and their investment in sophisticated calculations of networks of association between SNPs as meaningful markers of variation, lays the ground for an open-ended or 'open dataset', as Dana Greenfield (2016: 133) puts it, in which risks no longer silhouette the individual against the background mass of a population, but facilitate an interoperable negotiation of tensions around propensities, trains, descent, lineages and risks. Data is always partial, and an 'open data set' can be joined together with other data sets, some coming from other biosensors, some coming from completely different sources (social media, consumption habits).

The interpretation of DNA genotyping is complicated and has been understood in recent social research in different ways. In their account of 23andMe testing, Anna Harris, Susan Kelly and Sally Wyatt consider several major dimensions of the multiplication of tests associated with DNA biosensing. Their account of 'cybergenetics', or the intersection of genetic tests with social media, addresses perhaps the most prominent aspect of DNA biosensing: its mode of existence on Internet platforms. In their comprehensive mapping of the inception, popularisation, controversies and implications of DTC genetic tests, Harris and her co-authors emphasise both the new forms of agency associated with the tests – their term for this is 'autobiology', with its connotation of autobiography carried out through biology – and their inevitable exposure and complicity with forms of commodification and marketisation of scientific knowledge. They focus on a specific problem that arises in the convergence of genetic testing and Internet-based platforms – 'intersecting determinisms' – genetic determinism and a particularly prevalent technological determinism associated with the Internet: 'Our assumption is that determinisms of genetics are converging with determinisms of the internet, and from this convergence, genetic testing products have been developed, with internet-enabled reach directly to potential consumers and research participants far beyond the clinic' (Harris et al, 2016: 15).

Harris, Kelly and Wyatt track the genetic–Internet intersection by exploring autobiologies in the form of YouTube testimonials and the many blog and online community discussions of 23andMe results. They pay attention to the ways in which the 23andMe Internet platform has drawn on all the affordances and processes of recent social media to engage, enrol and maintain people in contact with the platform and its services, all the while constituting a body of data whose value takes the form of a product of research subjects who can be used for further scientific studies (we return to this topic later).

Harris and her co-authors conclude that the primary social reality of 23andMe genetic testing is a form of platform-enabled participation:

> 23andMe uses various internet platforms to construct an 'empowering' participatory culture, drawing on the democratising potential of the internet and personal genomics. 23andMe attempts to slip effortlessly between commercial and gift exchange, between selling a service and encouraging, even celebrating, research participation. The consumer-participant is presented as offering a saliva sample and personal information in exchange for gifts. (Harris et al, 2016: 91)

They analyse YouTube videos of test 'unboxing' or reading the test results as forms of autobiological participation. This mode of participation differs markedly from patients in states of illness, for whom test results have a quite different burden of expectation. The playful and curious engagements of YouTube videos, sometimes encouraged and certainly affirmed by

Figure 3.2: Close family tree, 23andMe Share and Compare

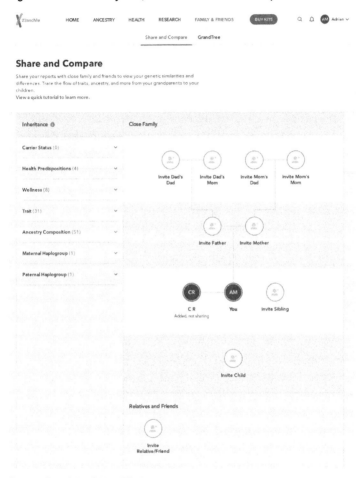

23andMe, epitomise Internet determinism or the belief that participation in the Internet is a practice of freedom. They are complemented, and in the last five years supplanted, by the participatory mechanisms engineered into 23andMe itself as an Internet platform.

On 23andMe, participation takes the form of 'sharing' (John, 2013). For example, on the login home page, under the title 'What you can do', users can select the option 'Share and Compare' and a pop-up window appears:

Please be thoughtful with sharing your insights. Share and Compare allows you to explore shared relationships and genetics. There is always the chance that you could learn something about yourself or your family that could be upsetting. Please be sensitive to others' right to choose for themselves whether they would like to know this kind of information. (23andMe, 2018e)

Agreeing to be thoughtful allows entry to the 'Share and Compare' page showing a close family tree (parents, grandparents, partners, siblings and children), not unlike the family tree we showed to our citizens' panel members. Unlike our scenario tree, the close family tree is hyperlinked to a survey page. Upon clicking on 'invite partner', for instance, the platform generates a new page 'Tell us about your partner' (23andMe, 2018e) (note that the URL for this page carries the words 'manage' and 'spouse', coding the close family differently to 'invite' and 'partner'). A series of questions unfold from this injunction: requests for names, permission to invite and a list of other possible connections who might be invited. These pages are typical of the ongoing enrolment and elicitation operating on the 23andMe platform. On almost any visit to the site as a logged-in user, further encouragements and inducements to share or invite other people appear. (For instance, 'trace the flow of DNA from grandparents to grandchildren in your family' suggests the possibility of tracing what is inherited cross-generationally, as long as four grandparents, two parents and their children all buy 23andMe tests.)

We can understand the frequent, recurrent elicitation of data from 23andMe users in several different ways. Harris and co-authors construe the Internet-boosted promise of participation as a thinly disguised attempt to gather more client data. 23andMe and the variety of other projects that solicit donations or the 'sharing' of genotyping data certainly do play on the now-almost-defunct register of Internet democracy. We contend that this experience of participation, however, is not merely a facade designed to simulate something that does not really exist. The elicitation of the responses has real 'network effects', in the same way that the many interactions we have with social media platforms have real effects on our lives when unexpected connections, contagions or responses arise in the wake of a posting. By virtue of their connective, associative architectures and practices, social media platforms intensify network effects. As Nick Srnicek (2016: 45) puts it 'the more numerous the users who use a platform, the more valuable that platform becomes for everybody else'.[8]

Although all social media platforms rely on network effects, 23andMe relies on it in a particularly focused way: social networks, especially networks that include family groups, change the significance of previously collected genotype data. They not only expand the scope and completeness of the ancestry-related information that might be provided to individuals ('trace the flow of DNA'), but also open up the possibility of conducting more targeted genotypical analyses of risks in the light of family traits and medical and health histories. Given that all genotyping implicitly compares an individual to a group or population,

---

[8]   When social science research literature first appeared on DTC genetic tests around 2008, it described a range of different tests. The fact that 23andMe and perhaps ubiome are the sole remaining competitors could be seen as a result of the network effects. Once one network begins to capture the relations between people, its network becomes disproportionately more valuable in comparison to others. As Srnicek (2016: 95) writes, 'with network effects, a tendency towards monopolisation is built into the DNA of platforms: the more numerous the users who interact on a platform, the more valuable the entire platform becomes for each one of them'.

any data that augments the variables or observations describing a population further the ongoing genotyping for individuals. From the perspective of scientists or others who analyse DNA data, the elicitation of further data from subjects augments the power and relevance of the data set in scientific terms, and this has direct relevance to the question of value around biosensing in a wider setting. From the perspective of the 'customers', once DNA biosensing comes to inhabit a platform setting such as 23andMe, it shifts into continuous gathering mode, not unlike that of tracking or monitoring forms of biosensing. The more people return to the platform, and the more they sign in to the platform, the more the data set around them grows and takes on significance and value for them (and others). For some people, questions or surveys that might not have held much interest before they received their test results and first reports might become interesting or relevant, for instance, after they find that their risk for age-related macular degeneration is slightly elevated.

Box 3.1: Making sense of genetic susceptibilities

By Mette Kragh-Furbo

My PhD research explored sense-making data practices in consumer genomics. By observing a subsection of an online forum for people living with a chronic illness and who undertake genetic testing to better understand and treat their illness, I found that sense-making is very much an embodied practice, where knowing your risks comes to matter practically. This is a sense-making practice that is not necessarily 'empowering' in the way imagined by consumer genomics companies like 23andMe. Instead, sense-making emerges as an ongoing, improvised and contingent practice of sharing and negotiating, discussing and figuring out, an embodied practice of translation characterised by confusion, struggle and uncertainty, but also hope and excitement. On the subsection of the forum that I observed, individuals share, discuss and negotiate their genetic susceptibilities, in particular, a number of SNPs that are considered relevant to decreased methylation. Methylation is a critical bodily process that regulates gene expression and builds neurotransmitters to process hormones, build immune cells, synthesise DNA and RNA, and process chemicals and toxins. Methylation reactions are important to the metabolism of nutrients, and it is believed by some alternative health practitioners, in particular, that the process can be compromised by medications, environmental toxicity and genetics. The theory of decreased methylation and its possible implications for health is an emerging knowledge, yet it is central to the discussions on the subsection of the forum. It is particularly discussed in relation to suggested treatment protocols that focus on adjusting diet and taking health supplements.

In their discussions of genetics and methylation, the individuals on the forum will draw on websites of medical professionals and alternative health practitioners, public databases such as PubMed, OMIN and dbSNP, and online encyclopaedias such as Wikipedia and SNPedia. Excerpts from a diversity of sources are shared and discussed in an effort to work out how to make sense of their genetic data and of their own illness symptoms. This is done in combination with spreadsheets and online analysis applications that are used to translate their 'raw' genetic data into risk profiles. For example, a freely available online application such as Strategene (Lynch, 2019) or GeneGenie can be used to analyse 'raw' 23andMe genetic data to provide information on specific SNPs that are considered relevant to methylation.

Some SNPs will be marked as mutated, partly mutated or unmutated. Associated discussion forums and information sheets advise on ways of addressing mutations. Yet, what does it mean to have a mutated copy of COMT V158M? And how do you address this mutation with health supplements? Together, the individuals on the forum are trying to work this out, yet this translation work is fraught with uncertainty and incompleteness. While it is possible to pay for 'interpretations' by using other online applications that will offer 'nutritional guides' and 'custom reports' (for example, LiveWello and Sterling's App from MTHFRsupport.com), my research shows that all of this translation work can only provide provisional directions that must be worked through in a process of 'trial and error'. Applications like these promise tailored (informational, not medical) advice, but individuals on the forum soon realise that such plans must be continuously negotiated and improvised, and that there is no personalised path, but only a process of personalising, always taking into account their own personal biographies and bodies. 'Go slow' is advice often repeated on the forum. This kind of biosensing practice requires careful and persistent 'body-work'. Genetic susceptibilities and supplement recommendations are put into practice and worked on in their incompleteness, only resolved momentarily. They can only provide partial clues for the caring of the unpredictable body, because when practising prediction, you always encounter instabilities, disruptions and ambivalence when making sense of the body. My research points towards a shift away from knowing about susceptibilities as advocated by consumer genomics companies like 23andMe, to living with susceptibilities that involve going beyond the susceptibility susceptible body of personalised medicine. Instead, knowing your risks becomes an embodied practice where the chronically ill body meets the susceptible body and the biochemical body in a kind of collective self-experimentation that is imbued with ambivalence and uncertainty, as well as hope and promise.

The value of *n* = 1 versus *n* = many

An account of 23andMe and similar enterprises that confines itself to the critique of platform-centred consumerism might miss the full range of biosensing propensities. Rightly, Harris and co-authors ask, as did the members of our citizens' panel, who might benefit from participation? Furthermore, why has collective ownership of data not taken hold? The account of the construction of an 'empowering' participatory culture that Harris and other recent work attributes to 23andMe does not allow room for the emergence of marginal biosensings. Our study of more distributed Internet-enabled DNA genotyping addressed how online groups collectively expanded their understanding of the SNP data supplied by 23andMe to include biological processes beyond the traits reported in the DTC test suite. The individual consumer, the form of self whose risks, traits, susceptibilities and propensities can be typed through genetic test, might change in the collective sensing of methylation. The 'auto' of autobiology has no fixed form when it comes to health understood in the broad sense of the capacity to react.

In their account of data citizens, Judith Gregory and Geoffrey Bowker (2016) sketch some elementary traits of a form of citizenship that might overflow the configured consumer. They start from the position that DNA biosensing data has a latent commonality or intrinsic sharedness. Given that all genotype data refers to a group, the primary process of genotyping is collective. Citizenship, Gregory and Bowker

Figure 3.3: Treatment of 23andMe SNP data

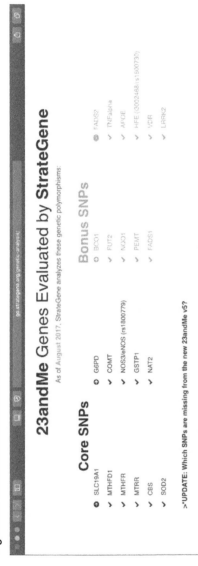

Source: Copyright of Dr Ben Lynch

(2016: 222) argue, takes root in this elementary feature of the data:

> If the notion of the "data citizen" suggests that data are always, in a sense, already "shared," then there is also a vast opportunity to create design spaces for individuals, social circles, health and medical fields, biosciences, scientific discovery. This design for novel design spaces could consider, but not be limited to, cross-sensory surrounds and affordances such as synaesthesia, artful abstraction, visual elegance and visible language, aural sensation and subtleties of sound, the tactile, the poetic, interactive vignettes that can be personalized, tales from the future, epistolary and otherwise, mindfulness, restfulness, peacefulness, wisdom-enhancing. In brief, the conditions of possibility exist to design for new digital literacies in shared data.

The notion of a data citizen shifts the register in which data maps self. Data, in its ongoing, expanding and transforming associations, becomes in this rendering a constitutive part of the citizen. We become citizens, Gregory and Bowker (2016: 214) suggest, because we are 'saturated by data flows, markers, indicators, analyses' that we cannot ignore because they vitally concern us. This is almost the first lesson of the genetic tests in their multiplication: the flood of associations between different parts of genomes and the many conditions and traits, the manifold attempts to expand the explanatory power of the patterns of associations by differentiating groups and populations, and the lived and embodied histories of exposures and environments (the 'exposome' as Gregory and Bowker term it) render it almost impossible to keep the boundaries of an individual, inscribed in their 'biology', intact. Gregory and Bowker start from the position that the data is likely, like biology, to be commensal and parasitic, or even completely ecological in its overflows and entanglements. The fact that we experience great uncertainty about what data to share – our citizens' panel frequently mentioned this, and every sign-in to 23andMe brings with it a renewed sense of this difficulty – does not mean that sharing is both primary and problematic. Just as the GWAS track epistemically unstable associations between variations in DNA, the sharing of data through hybrid social–corporate–clinical platforms seeds problematic but potentially generative associations between individuals.

Given that biosensing practices often circulate data as part and parcel of the process of understanding, the question is: how could circulation occur in ways that augment senses of common ownership rather than instilling a sense of its loss or forfeit to aggressively capitalising platforms? The consumer-side platform interfaces of 23andMe present a lopsided view of the circulation of data. Much of the appearance, interactivity and user interface design of 23andMe frames the individual consumer as the endpoint of DNA tests, as the knowledgeable, risk-aware, choice-making agent, piloting their health trajectory.

The platform architecture and its scaffolding of scientific knowledge infrastructure and work (GWAS) has another less prominent but no less vital aspect. On this side of the platform, DNA genotyping tests contribute to a mass archive of biomedical cases whose value lies in the aggregate and in their potential for further research. The sense-making taking place on this side of the platform is much more open-ended and diffuse, but it lends itself to work that transforms senses of self. Like the para-platform and para-clinical settings that Kragh-Furbo explores in functional disorders, the ongoing scientific work provides the necessary condition for the platform to capitalise on the future value of the data. The scientific work overflows the platform-user framing, and this overflow could be immensely important in doing DNA biosensing differently. 23andMe's own scientific publications (23andMe, 2018c) attest to the significance of the scientific side of the platform. The publications stem from collaborations between the company and biomedical researchers in universities and drug companies (for an example collaboration between 23andMe and GlaxoSmithKline, see Ehm et al, 2017).

For an individual 23andMe user who has consented to the use of their data in research, the path followed by their data can be difficult to track. As the 'Research' pages on 23andMe observe: 'On average, a customer who chooses to opt into research contributes to over 230 studies on topics that range from Parkinson's disease to lupus to asthma and more' (23andMe, 2018d).

Some of these studies combine the architecture of the genotyping platform with other biosensing platforms. Studies on asthma conducted in collaboration with Mt Sinai Hospital or on heart health with Stanford University, for instance, involve apps on iPhones that track steps and movement, as well as periodic surveys, to generate data that will be merged with the genotype data from the microarrays so that 'you can help drive scientific and medical discoveries' (23andMe, 2018d). In these cases, data flows across platforms and biosensors embedded in other devices such as smartphones. The 23andMe platform becomes what Plantin et al (2016) describe as an interconnected system of parts, acting as a seamless whole. This platform is a proliferation of connections: 'Genetics for Your App', suggests 23andMe (2018b) in announcing the availability of genotyping data through an online programmable interface (the Application Programme Interface [API]) that can be integrated in apps or other websites.

It is difficult to determine exactly how financially valuable the 23andMe data set is. After recent growth in North America and Europe, purchases of genetic and ancestry testing kits total more than five million (Kennett, 2018; Regalado, 2018). The genotyping data spans nations and geographies, and as a data set, it remains open on all sides to further growth (for example, new reports arise from reanalysis of existing data in the light of newly published scientific studies). It is very likely that the 23andMe business model concerns the collected data, not the genetic tests.

The crowdsourcing of data is at the core of the platform. Almost everything that customers encounter when they log in to the site and explore it concerns the accretion and refining of those data. As Gregory and Bowker (2016: 218) observe: 'if you look at their practices, many actually don't interact with their data very much or very often. That's why we need to understand practices, not only expressed opinions, to get at what people are actually doing'.

What people are actually doing with genotype data involves a range of platform practices without a central point of reference. Although it is difficult to gauge proportions, some people move their data away from the genetic test platform. Discussions in online forums such as Reddit (see: www.reddit.com/r/23andme or www.reddit.com/r/snpedia), as well as the 'community' forums on 23andMe and other DNA testing sites, suggest lively interest in expanding the significance of the data, particularly in relation to kinship and ancestry. Popular threads on Reddit discuss how to identify birth kin ('find my real father') using genomics and genealogy websites such as GEDmatch.com, dna.land or Ancestry.com. Although ethnicity and kinship discussions are most common, disease, weight, exercise, diet and longevity are common topics. Even if people might not interact with their data very much (How many times a month does an average 23andMe user sign in to their account after the initial excitement about the test results have worn off?), their data might be interacting without them. Contributing 'on average … to over 230 studies', their data also changes their association with others.

The data citizen, if we follow Gregory and Bowker's account, does not depend on a self–other boundary. A data citizen is, in their terms, attuned to what is collective or associative in data, especially in the distributed institutional knowledge-power arrangements of health, education and work. DNA biosensing, despite the bright design of 'the new you' on the genotyping platforms, intimates another actuality, a more distributed sense of self.

Radical data dividuation

Dana Greenfield (2016) has begun to articulate the conceptual underpinnings of data citizenship in her analysis of Quantified Self (QS) practices. She targets the statistics of $n = 1$, or the idea that an individual's data could be the basis of interpretation. In classical statistics, a data set of $n = 1$ concerns only one subject. Given that statistics studies the properties of populations, an $n = 1$ data set has no statistical value. In a well-sampled population, n should be a significant proportion of the total population. Yet, in QS practices, and we suggest, DNA biosensing, $n = 1$ data practices come to matter.

In contrast to the individualising promise of many DNA genotyping products, Greenfield's account of $n = 1$ modes of data interpretation hinges on dividuation:

> The pixelated n of 1 is a subject ever divided into finer granularity, but also whose partial datasets can be joined with others, in networked, dividuated in data. The individual is no longer cast against and modelled alongside the mass; rather the *crowd* and the n of 1 melt into each other. In other words, the crowd or open data set anticipated an n of 1 that is already pixelated, made of similar stuff to the crowd, "interoperable" data points to be seamlessly joined to the *n of billions/billion 1s*. (Greenfield, 2016: 133)

In this passage, 'pixelated' refers to any rendering of a person or subject in data. Greenfield outlines several related trajectories for subjects 'dividuated in data': precision medicine's intensification of the personal; 'tracking for self-care' working against rigid clinical or medical categorisations; and 'living the data stream' rendering experience through data and narrative. Dividuated subjects have less decisive agency than that attributed to consumers. They live in the midst of incomplete and changing data sets and constructs of their relatedness. The growth of ancillary DNA genotyping analysis platforms such as SNPedia, codegen, DNA.Land (DNA.LAND, 2018), Genes for Good (GenesForGood, 2018) and Promethease marks how relations between individuals and populations are rewired. Clinical or scientific statements of risk or susceptibility, as we have seen, locate individuals within a population distribution. 'Pixelated' – that is, constitutively datafied – subjects explore the variations of curves of relatedness ranging across health, disease, ancestry/genealogy, kinship and ethnicity.

With the advent of whole genome sequencing services such as Genos (Genos, 2018), in which the range of variations and connections to scientific literature extends well beyond the GWAS underpinnings of 23andMe, the ecology of crowd-mediated data points is likely to expand. These services encompass many other forms of DNA variation beyond SNPs. New kinds of variations will be ingested by analysis services such as Promethease. Greenfield (2016: 126) suggests that the $n = 1$ should be understood as 'an experimental system where new possibilities for the meaning and experience of health and illness ramify in surprising ways'. Even if $n = 1$ remains subject to capture in high-end personalised medicine, the growth of a crowd of $n = 1$s is somewhat different since it comprises a matrix of partial views. It enables 'a different form of medical knowledge production, it refuses the logics of scale, aggregation and standardization' (Greenfield, 2016: 136), redirecting data towards a zone of group, self and kin determinations.

Conclusions

DNA biosensing is not a simple practice. As we have seen, DNA genotyping departs from tests of genomic variations (SNPs).

Only some variations can be framed as health risks. Although patterns of variations can be associated with risks and disease susceptibilities, the tests observe many variations at the same time. In relation to health, DNA biosensing operates largely in a promissory mode, feeding into open-ended and expanding data sets whose biomedical significance awaits confirmation through further research. Beginning with the design of the microarray device (the biosensor) and running through to the analysis and reanalysis of the data, DNA biosensing relies on the ongoing production of large-scale scientific studies of genomic variations, especially in the form of the thousands of GWAS. Like DNA itself, genotyping shows an extraordinary mutability and variability in its own right. It addresses seemingly every aspect of identity and agency, collective and individual: behaviour, kinship, intelligence, appearance, political preferences run alongside many physiological and metabolic traits. As scientific knowledge changes, genotyping and its significance alters. Although DNA biosensors do not (yet) offer the continuous stream of sensing associated with some other biosensors discussed in this book, DNA biosensing absorbs some of the scientific publications, findings and data that constantly appear in these fields. It effectively operates as a stream.

Like parcels from Amazon, DNA kits for health and ancestry testing owe their existence to the logistics of Internet platforms and their entry into the everyday. Platforms coordinate and mediate people's engagement with DNA biosensing both in measuring and in analysing, and, perhaps most importantly, as configured contributors of data to databases that support further research. People's position in relation to the platforms is not simple. Social-scientific accounts of the tests reflect that complexity. They sometimes describe the construction of the engaged, participatory consumer of the tests as an artifice to collect data. Arrangements for participation rely on platform interactivity and sociality, especially around kinship and ongoing research. The platforms actually mediate between multiple groups. Researchers themselves have been configured as consumers of platform-generated data sets. The architecture of the platforms largely confirms the primacy of markets as the social ordering practice.

From the standpoint of biosensing as a practice, the tests and analysis of them overflow any simple account of consumption. A proliferation of hand-crafted, special-purpose or public workflows and pipelines for the exploration of data offers one sign of this overflow. Ideas of the 'data citizen' and $n = 1$ proposed in some accounts, as well as some aspects of the notion of 'autobiology', begin to move in different directions. They expand well beyond clinical genetics' assessment of disease risks. They diverge from the institutionally affirmed vision of personalised predictive medicine pursued by biomedical research. They percolate into collective practices of living with illness or other health conditions.

4

Biosensing in Old Age

Remote care or care at a distance for older people has been developing in discursive contexts that tap into the dual tropes of ageing as a social problem or burden resulting in a 'care crisis' (Matthews-King, 2018), and older people as intrinsically at risk (Pickard, 2009). Yet, older people are not necessarily sick, or not sick enough, for the ageing body to be brought into the clinic. The professionally adopted shift from chronological to functional definitions of ageing and the notion of the life course have come to underpin the character and organisation of care for older people, who are increasingly subject to 'techniques of measurement, standardisation and intervention' (Marshall and Katz, 2016: 146). With population ageing often framed as an economic burden, older people considered to be frail find themselves in a preclinical space, a kind of waiting room serviced by sensors and systems of monitoring. It is in this waiting room that we have observed forms of telecare playing a role, or attempting to facilitate 'care' rather than medicine.

Sensor-based home monitoring, or 'telecare' as it is often termed, differs, on the face of it, from the examples of biosensing that we have so far examined in this book. Within this field, there is, of course, a spectrum of domestic monitoring systems and devices that fall broadly into health-related and care-oriented modes. In the health/medical mode, 'telehealth' systems aim to improve 'patient activation' or self-care, providing users with readings of vital signs and facilitating the uploading or transmitting of data about their bodies for consideration by professionals. In contrast, the 'care' mode includes automated movement and home environment sensors that send signals to remote monitoring centres and usually trigger a phone call back to the 'user'; these are most usually referred to as 'telecare' rather than 'telehealth'. While many sensor-based devices collect data from the body for interpretation, in home telecare, there is less emphasis on the active self-tracking of health and more on the preservation of an existing state or 'safety', the maintenance of a kind of waiting, seen in many examples of monitoring systems generating automated messages about (it is claimed) bodily states.

However, one feature that telecare systems have in common with other biosensors explored in this book is the attempt to simplify and address what are inherently complex and often recalcitrant body states or situations. As we shall see, this attempt at simplification is also connected with the broader imaginary of redefining care as a commodity to be purchased (either privately or by the state), and of monitoring and managing large numbers of 'problematic' older people and automating aspects of care through forms of assemblage or platforms. A home telecare system attempts to connect an older person's body/bodily state with devices such as a fall detector, door exit sensor, medication dispenser and so on, as can be seen in the example in Figure 4.1. In turn, messages or data produced connect with a range of others: call centre, family, care services and so on.

The promise held out by telecare takes many forms. In the health mode, promises include education of the user about particular health conditions, in which the person is usually identified as a patient who has a particular diagnosis, with the explicit aim of preventing hospital admission.[1] The claimed

---

[1] Many high-profile, funded trials have been conducted to examine the effect of such systems on hospital admission and the use of health services and drugs, such as the Whole Systems Demonstrator (see Steventon et al, 2013; Henderson et al, 2014) and the LCIA Test Bed (see: www.lciatestbed.org.uk), but none have so far provided conclusive evidence of effectiveness in those terms.

Figure 4.1: Tunstall home emergency response

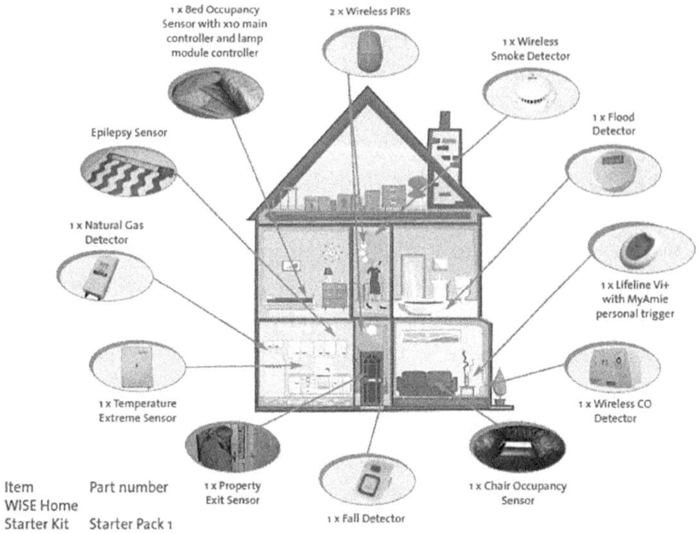

Item WISE Home Starter Kit — Part number: Starter Pack 1

Source: Copyright of Tunstall Healthcare (UK), Ltd

benefits include affording people greater involvement in, and therefore responsibility for, their long-term conditions as in the following example from Philips (2018):

Empower chronic patients with better self-care approaches

The eCAC ambulatory telehealth program gives care teams the capability to monitor and coach high-risk chronic patients, helping them improve their ability to manage their own condition. Guidelines-based care plans are tailored for the unique needs of each patient, delivering a personalized experience for patients while enabling care teams to scale their efforts.

However, in the care mode, and where the condition is ageing rather than sickness, systems are shaped towards the remote management and monitoring of a person, in which they are identified as a recipient of care, at risk and, in many ways, problematic. Here, the promises include preventing admission to long-term residential care. The claimed benefits include 'peace of mind' and maintenance of 'independence' at home for those people considered frail or vulnerable, usually because they are very old or suffer from forms of dementia, as in the following example from Tunstall (2018b):

Solutions for Social Care

Our Connected Care solutions have been designed to support a wide range of people, including older people, people at risk of falls, people with limited mobility, people with learning disabilities, people with dementia and people with conditions such as epilepsy.

Some forms of telecare involve continuous monitoring; others function intermittently. Analogue falls detectors (currently using landline telephones) are socially highly significant given the rapidly increasing numbers of frail older people to whom they become attached in the UK. They are also attempting to capture bodily states that scroll through almost infinite variations. Perhaps monitoring the body's movements can be just as tricky as measuring the body's internal flows and processes (hormones/genes)? Furthermore, just as knowing about your chances of getting Alzheimer's disease through direct-to-consumer genetic testing, and the management of anxiety for couples trying to conceive through ovulation-monitoring devices, the falls detector is being marketed as a key component of managing risk. Yet, as we shall see, calculating what is and is not a fall turns out to defy even the smartest of detectors.

Self-tracking or dys-tracking?

Within the growing literature on self-tracking, the quantification of the body and, to some extent, digital health, most research attention has been paid to those health-tracking devices, such as the Fitbit, predominantly, but not exclusively, marketed at well-resourced young and middle-aged consumers. Marshall and Katz (2016) note that this research literature has neglected ageing, and we agree. Our studies of local authority-provided telecare for older people in Northshire UK, shows the proliferation of those telecare devices such as chair and bed occupancy sensors that reach far into the home, monitoring everyday actions and sometimes intimate spaces of people's lives. As we have noted (for example, Roberts et al, 2012; Atkinson, 2019), such monitoring also reaches into people's embodied sense of self and can reshape what 'care' means and involves. Assessed as at risk, the recipient of telecare is configured as having little agency, while it follows that the remote monitoring centre works in responsive, rather than social or even therapeutic, mode. A common telecare device, the falls detector, for example, is designed not to educate, self-track or promote healthier behaviours, but instead to keep the older (defined as vulnerable) person 'safe' – to manage risk. Katz and Marshall (2018: 65) have noted 'a differentiation of wearable tracking technologies that replicate[s] a cultural separation of subject bodies into, on the one hand, those which are risk-averse/independent/active and, on the other hand, those which are risk-prone/dependent/passive'. Indeed, it is not the devices that are active or passive, but the bodies/persons inscribed in them.

In contrast with the projection of many biosensors as self-trackers, we propose that many telecare devices represent not so much self-tracking as *dys-tracking*. Automated falls detectors do not require anything of the wearer except the wearing and perhaps, if possible, a verbal response to the alarm call that sounds through the home-installed hub unit. How have we got to this point? The oldest and most common form of telecare is the (wearer-activated) red button pendant alarm worn around the neck in the home. This device is self-activated: the wearer presses the button if they feel they need help and the call centre is alerted. This form of telecare has remained popular, but it is known that the majority of pendant wearers fail to press the button when they fall; it seems 'users' either simply do not connect a fall with the action of pressing the red button or express reluctance to disturb relatives or the emergency services (Fleming and Brayne, 2008). This finding partly prompted the introduction of a separate but linked device, the falls detector, which could activate automatically. These devices draw on accelerometer technology to sense changed body angle, speed of fall and air pressure in order to determine that a person has fallen. Whatever agency resided in the pendant button arrangement was delegated to an accelerometer.[2] In the falls detectors in large-scale current use, it is a change in the body/position of the body that sets off the alarm – or not, as the case may be, as detectors often only register 'hard falls', a problem that is recognised from within the industry (Doris, 2014; see also later).

Initially, we thought about the term 'dys-tracking' as connoting the passive, disconnected, frail and vulnerable subject bodies to which, for example, falls detectors become attached and the shift from calling for help to help as triggered (or not, see later). However, dys-tracking may also have resonance here in the sense of consciousness. For the most part, wearers of the Fitbit or OV-Watch Fertility Predictor, for example, are consciously tracking themselves, that is, their vital signs or ovulation patterns. Self-consciously adopted fitness trackers such as 'Moov Now' arguably provide a form of data that can allow for comparisons with the efforts and achievements of others (albeit along with the harvesting of data to be utilised commercially).

---

[2] A telecare system as a whole may include a number of linked automated devices installed such as a smoke detector, gas detector, flood detector, enuresis sensor, door exit sensor, medication dispenser and so on.

Measurements can be used interactively: some older people wearing Fitbits discuss the resulting data with others and thus enhance social interactions (Katz and Marshall, 2018). Contrast this with a very different kind of biosensor, the falls detector, and dys-tracking comes to mean (being subject to) a remote observation, promoted as affording a level of peace of mind both for the wearer and distant others. Of course, this is not to say that some 'users'[3] may not have voluntarily agreed to wear such a monitor, and that some may understand how it works and what it does and does not provide, but the constituency at which it is primarily aimed (frail older people assessed as low functioning) are the least likely to be wearing this consciously or voluntarily, as we have shown (Mort et al, 2013; Atkinson, 2019). Most recently, we asked one older person about the (falls detector) device around her wrist: "I don't know about it, I don't know what it's for dear" (wearer, falls monitor, August 2018).

The struggle to make sense of falls and telecare data

Again, while self-tracking devices such as Fitbits promise some greater self-knowledge through knowing your metrics, what kind of metrics are/can be produced from automatic monitoring systems? Apart from ethical issues around who owns and uses any forthcoming 'data', there is a question about what is, or can be learned from, for example, a frail older person's movement around the house. It seems that the platformisation of telecare is less advanced than other forms of biosensing. Although the analogue devices such as falls detectors are one element in an assemblage of people, skills, buildings and communication networks, and thus are platformed, they are not part of digitally aggregating large numbers of data points. This is largely because most forms of telecare, often termed 'first generation' and

[3]   Along with others, for example, Suchman (2002), we have critiqued the term 'user' in the telecare context (Mort et al, 2013).

exemplified by the pendant alarm, have existed for more than 30 years, and many of these are still in use and problematic to replace. In the context of public provision, the digitisation of telecare systems is restricted by austerity measures, but also by ethical concerns about privacy and confidentiality.

So-called second-generation telecare systems such as 'Just Checking' (see Figure 4.2), however, are platforms designed for family members/carers and professionals. Patterns of movement can be collected online over period of, say, two months, which can then, it is claimed, inform highly significant decisions about care needs and provision, such as whether the older person does or does not need to go into residential care. In this case, the system is designed so that data can be analysed within a small community of users such as family, possibly with named professionals, to inform decisions, and such systems can be purchased privately or publicly.

It is worth asking what benchmark or version of movement activity is considered outside of normal for older people living at home who are subject to dys-tracking devices, an issue that has also been raised in relation to the self-tracking ones (Crawford et al, 2015). Using functionality as the primary means of measuring ageing has been heavily criticised as enhancing the pathologisation of old age, as Oxlund and Whyte (2014) detail in their review article. In exploring local authority-commissioned telecare in the UK, we found little, if any, attempt to learn from available quantitative data about call frequency or call attribution, let alone patterns of movement. This implies a view of the 'telecare user' as beyond therapy and unable to interact meaningfully with the installed system. This public provision, such as in Northshire, is a responsive, rather than proactive, service, an ironic exception being that those clients who triggered an excessive number of calls were considered problematic, requiring additional assessment (Mort et al, 2013). Issues of social class and inequality are, we suggest, also prominent here: most of the telecare services that we

Figure 4.2: The Just Checking system

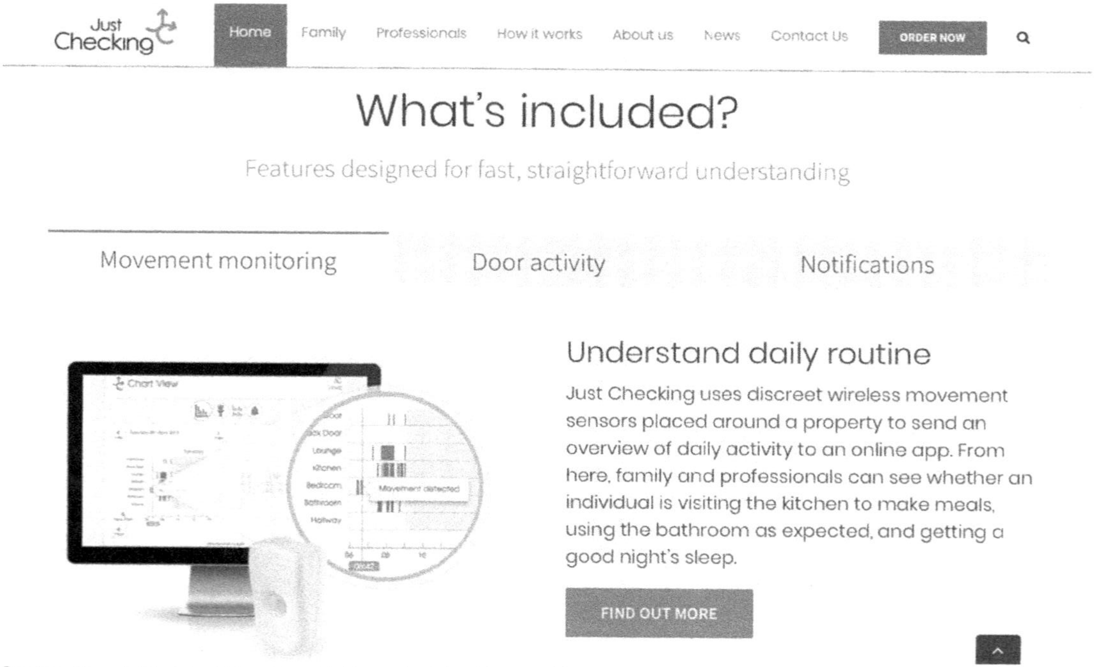

Source: Copyright of Just Checking, Ltd (www.justchecking.co.uk)

studied were prescribed at no cost to people living with very low incomes, with the clearly stated aim of reducing admissions to publicly financed aged-care facilities. The frail users of telecare in Northshire are a long way from the empowered, wealthy self-trackers figured in the original call from Intel Labs for research proposals mentioned in the Preface.

In contrast to telehealth applications such as blood glucose/diabetes monitoring, the potential for harvesting big data from publicly provided telecare services seems to have, as yet, been accorded little importance. Analysis of patterns of telecare use at either the individual or regional scale would require the allocation of extra resources, and in the UK context of austerity in public policy and provision, this seems unlikely. In a context in which domestic spaces are increasingly populated by (privately purchased) data-gathering Internet-connected devices such as televisions, energy meters and so-called 'smart speakers' like Amazon's Alexa and Google Home (which use machine learning to detect patterns of activity and content of speech), this apparent lack of interest in the data generated by telecare devices seems anomalous, even anachronistic. Perhaps it will ultimately be the corporations who sell telecare systems to local authorities who will think of ways to generate profit from analysing the captured data? We can imagine scenarios where care providers could try to tweak their face-to-face services based on information about the sleeping and movement patterns of older people living at home, for example, although this would create ethical problems in a (publicly funded) care context. In addition, analysing telecare usage becomes very difficult if most calls are false alarms or test calls. Furthermore, as we shall see, it is extremely hard to make sense of the data provided by falls detectors, in particular, because some falls are undetectable. What degree of accuracy could be obtained when a 'soft fall' may not be registered? In this sense, currently applied forms of telecare arguably constitute 'un-smart' surveillance, rather than the provision of intelligence about a person's home activity patterns.

Crawford et al (2015) are also concerned with issues of agency and power in their comparative study of wearable self-tracking devices and the development of the weight scale. As a stand-alone device, the weight scale, which began life in public places as the 'penny scale', has found its way into domestic bathrooms and provides self-knowledge and promotes fitness. However, it is up to the user whether they wish to share their weight reading with others. By contrast, the Microsoft Band or the Jawbone UP, among others, allow the user to view their data, but these are also harvested by the company and may also be shared/sold to third-party analytics companies. The telecare falls detectors and door exit sensors, in contrast, track body movements in order to trigger an alarm and, in this way, provide information (if largely incoherent) to others, but they offer no self-knowledge or opportunity for improvement. The falls monitor triggers an alarm and the possibility of a face-to-face response; it is sold as preventive, although it cannot prevent a fall. Ironically, the notorious number of false alarms triggered by falls devices impacts negatively when this creates and reinforces older people's perceptions of themselves as being frail, a nuisance and dependent.

Researching telecare in use

As we shape technologies, so we build society (Bijker and Law, 1994), but what chances do groups of older people and carers have to shape telecare systems and therefore society? This question, in particular, has informed both our citizens' panel approach to understanding telecare and our parallel ethnographic observations of telecare in use.[4] Insights from both approaches are given in Box 4.1.

---

[4] Our research has received a series of ethical approvals, including from Northshire Council Research Ethics Committee and Lancaster University Research Ethics Committee. The team has been covered throughout by relevant Disclosure and Barring Service, and previously Criminal Records Bureau, checks.

Box 4.1: Falls detectors in social care

By Theresa Atkinson

I have followed the implementation of Northshire Council's redesigned telecare service, mapping, observing and analysing telecare work in action, in practice, exploring everyday encounters with telecare. This ethnographic approach was unconstrained by what Pols (2012) argued to be one-dimensional standardised research designs, and examined how telecare was provided, experienced, evaluated and evidenced in what was a difficult and dynamic organisational use setting. My ethnographic work included: shadowing and observation; in-depth interviews and follow-ups with service users, carers, senior managers and social care staff; and the analysis of policy documents and monitoring centre data of telecare use at the point of 'activation'. While I examined everyday experiences with telecare, I also considered its consequences for the everyday lives of those older people who came to 'use', 'not use' or 'misuse' the system.

The Tunstall 'iVi' was a falls detection device in frequent use when I began my study. This device is usually worn around the neck, although it can also be clipped to clothing and worn as a brooch or fixed to a belt around the waist. The iVi has different movement sensors, from low to high, to reflect the different mobilities or immobilities of its potential users. The falls algorithm for the iVi is designed to detect changes in barometric pressure, acceleration and static orientation to assess whether a fall has taken place, although these types of devices do not necessarily detect a slow slide out of a chair or bed:

> The iVi intelligent pendant with automatic fall detection is a small body worn device that can be used to raise manual alarms by using the integral help button. The device can also detect falls and raise an automatic alarm using an integrated accelerometer and a barometer. The device is sealed to a rating of IP67, which means the device can be used in the bath/shower without causing an issue. The fall algorithm is designed to make use of changes in barometric pressure, acceleration and static orientation in order to assess whether a fall event has taken place.

> When the iVi detects an event which is assessed to be like a fall, (this takes up to 20 seconds) then it will alert the user by emitting tones from the sounder and lighting the green LED. The user then has 10 seconds to cancel the alert by pressing the cancel button. (Tunstall Group, 2018a)

In practice, though, this particular device was observed to be highly sensitive to everyday movement:

> "I realised like if I did something – and say you were in the kitchen and I dropped a spoon it would go off, so I stopped wearing that and I keep it by the locker." (Service user, July 2016).

> This service user had a history of falls and kept her iVi falls detector on her mantelpiece and she said that it was going off all the time. I picked it up and placed it in the palm of my hand turning it over gently and it immediately triggered a call to the call centre, unintentionally demonstrating its sensitivity. I gave it back to her and she put it back on the mantelpiece. (Field note, June 2016)

When the iVi was launched in 2013, there was speculation that it might replace the existing 'red button' alarms in use in the UK:

Automatic pendant could save NHS millions of pounds a year

> Tunstall has launched one of the world's most-sophisticated fall detection alarms that automatically calls for help in the event of a fall.

> The new iVi device, which is manufactured in the UK, could save hundreds of lives a year and the NHS millions of pounds.

> The automatic pendant offers an unprecedented detection algorithm that reacts to changes in barometric pressure, acceleration and static orientation and determines whether a fall has taken place. It is likely to replace tens of thousands of the 1.7 million 'red button' telecare pendants currently in use in the UK. (Building Better Healthcare, 2013)

However, because of uncertainties around what might constitute a fall, I observed some service users being advised locally to wear both devices (the fall detector and the red button alarm), even though the falls detectors had dual functionality with built-in manual and automatic triggering mechanisms, as well as a call-cancellation facility. The 'Vibby', the most recent falls detection device in use, was frequently worn around the wrist like an i-watch. The Vibby is promoted as a device that potentially reduces the number of false alarms. This is achieved, it is claimed, by detecting 'heavy' or 'serious' falls, with its detection attributes based on loss of altitude and acceleration. The Vibby, however, does not necessarily detect a 'soft' fall, particularly where a person holds on to something to slow down acceleration in an attempt to reduce the impact of a fall, so users are still being advised to wear both devices.

However, wearing different devices can not only be confusing, stigmatising and objectifying, but also indicate a lack of trust in the workability or effectiveness of the system:

> The Vibby was designed to pick up a fall automatically but the installer recommended that Margaret should also wear the red button alarm on her other wrist, as well as the falls device, so that she could choose which one to press if the falls detector failed to trigger an alarm in the event of a fall.... Margaret was confused about the instructions and about the Vibby's dual functionality and she questioned whether, when and in what circumstances it would work ... the installers often had difficulty demonstrating how the Vibby could trigger a call in the event of a fall. The installer, for example, attempted to demonstrate to Margaret how the Vibby worked and dropped it on the carpet to simulate a fall but the device didn't activate – she tried it twice and on the third occasion it triggered a call to the monitoring centre (another installer on a different occasion resorted to dropping the device in the lid of a cardboard box as the hard surface seemed to trigger an alert on the first attempt). (Field note, February 2017)

Many of the wearable 'automatic' falls-related devices were seemingly not very 'intelligent', sometimes being over- or under-sensitive in everyday use, only picking up certain types of falls, and not always able to distinguish between an actual 'fall' and a 'non-fall' situation:

> Reg described how he'd pulled a chest of drawers on top of himself, falling over in the process, but his 'intelligent' falls device failed to trigger an alert and he was told he should have pressed the button. Reg said that his device went off frequently, but not when he fell, but the 'false' calls gave him reassurance that 'someone' was there and he had regular unscheduled contact with the monitoring centre staff albeit via falsely activated calls. (Field note, May 2017)

Falls detectors sometimes generated a multitude of calls, and particularly false alarm calls. It is known that this often leads to the falls detectors being rejected (Igual et al, 2013). False calls (and it is not always that clear how they get recorded as such) can sometimes invade older people's privacy in multiple ways. Older people's movement, activity or inactivity in the home is being monitored/detected/ recorded/responded to, yet the majority of calls, including for falls monitoring, appear to be made for non-emergency use (Northshire, 2018) While falls monitoring can promote a sense of security (sometimes false), it can also create demand and dependency, and enhance older people's sense of vulnerability and fragility:

> Don't know why it's gone off; I just dropped it; Yes I'm ok – I'm just on the toilet; It went off – I just touched it; I'm ok but got something wrong with washing machine; ... are you on the floor ... the carer's coming; it's going off all the time – so he's taken it off; are you sitting on it?; she just wants her dinner; I'm hungry; I'm cold – it's freezing in here. (Field notes, May 2015, June 2017, July 2017)

> I wasn't sure whether Margaret (who had capacity and was physically active) was being reassured by the offer of telecare or whether it was making her feel more anxious.... I watched Margaret as she closed her eyes, and crossed her hands in front of her chest, as the installer reminded her about her potential vulnerabilities, about the risks of falling, in particular, but also about other risks from fire and poisonous gases as the installer checked the other devices – the smoke and CO_2 detectors which had been previously installed in her flat even though she had the ability to raise an alarm herself. (Field note, February 2017)

There was a significant increase in telecare installations once the service was introduced charge-free, including the use of wearable falls devices. Some older people did resist, and for multiple reasons; others never wore them or had never used them in an emergency, but nevertheless retained them for 'peace of mind'. Some also adapted the prescribed order of things and chose whether, when and what to use, choosing and controlling their own risks, determining which device or devices best suited their personal day-to-day needs. Some preferred a device such as the (active) pendant alarm, rather than devices that allow passive monitoring such as the 'automatic' falls detectors.

There are many different types of 'falls' and a diverse range of 'fallers'. There are numerous fall detectors, monitors and sensors, with multiple and heterogeneous contexts within which a 'fall' is experienced and situated. This makes detecting, monitoring and responding to a fall a complex, messy, unstable and unpredictable undertaking.

In Northshire, as in many other local authorities in the UK, the costs of providing social care have been escalating in conjunction with severe cuts in general budget allocations from central government. The decision to remove charges (previously a means-tested eligibility scale was applied) was prompted by two aspects of telecare experience: first, that uptake had been slow despite encouragement by social workers and others; and, second, that there remained a belief that at scale, the provision of remote care would result in significant savings in the adult social care spend due to a reduction in face-to-face homecare visits. We use the term 'belief' because the evidence available for such savings remains, at best, contradictory (Woolham et al, 2018).

Since charges were removed, the number of telecare installations in Northshire has escalated sharply (from about 1,000 to 10,000), with most systems being provided to older people living at home. In the majority of cases, the 'user' will be provided with a pendant or wrist-worn alarm, a linked smoke detector and, if assessed as at risk of falling, a falls detector, worn on the wrist or round the waist. As we have seen, because of uncertainties around what constitutes a 'fall' and around what can be detected by the device, some older people end up with two alarm systems, one of which has automated falls detection built in. It has yet to be determined whether Northshire Council has realised the expected savings, but the increase in telecare user numbers has allowed us to continue observing, with the appropriate consents, how systems are being experienced in the home.

Figure 4.3: The 'Vibby' fall detector

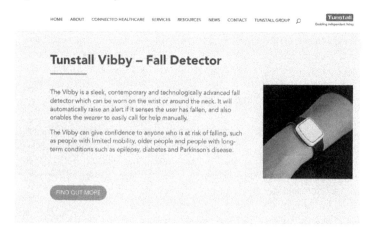

Source: Copyright of Tunstall Healthcare (UK), Ltd

Figure 4.4: Margaret wears both devices

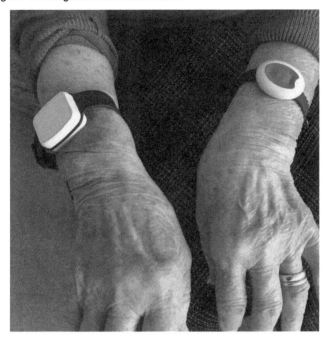

Citizens' (not patients' or service users') perspectives on sensor-based home care

Building on earlier work using citizens' juries and panels to assess community health needs or express views about the introduction of telemedicine (for example, Kashefi and Mort, 2004; Mort et al, 2009), between 2006 and 2011, Roberts, Milligan and Mort conducted a series of group discussions about telecare. We carried these out in a range of different settings and contexts to complement our observational ethnographic work in the UK. Held prior to our 2014 Intel-funded citizens' panel on genetic testing and ovulation biosensors (Mort et al, 2016), these meetings included: a disabled people's group; three older people's forums (consultative groups supported by local authorities); two carers' groups; and one Asian carers' forum. We convened citizens' panels in residential homes and also through continuing learners' groups at Lancaster University. These meetings formed part of the wider Ethical Frameworks for Telecare Technologies (EFORTT) FP7 project in which 22 citizens' panels on ethical aspects of remote care provision in four European Union (EU) countries were held (EFORTT Researchers, 2011; Milligan et al, 2011; Mort et al, 2015). The purpose was to provide a critical, deliberative axis for this research and to open up possibilities for older people to enter the policy debate around the changing nature of care and care work.

The panels began by discussing what the participants considered to be 'good care'. After that discussion, we showed panels a number of telecare devices and systems currently in use and invited responses about how and in what ways these might (or might not) contribute to 'good care' as defined by participants. A theme that emerged from many of these discussions was how the implementation of the remote monitoring of older people at home to keep them safe rendered many of the existing care and self-care practices of older people invisible – as if older people did nothing otherwise to ensure their own safety. At the end of one of these panel meetings, a participant passed us a note in which she described one of her own daily reciprocal care strategies (see Figure 4.5).

The note in Figure 4.5 serves to highlight all those often-undocumented activities in people's lives, often involving neighbours and friends, into which a sensor-based version of care gets introduced (Mort et al, 2013). It also shows how technological home risk monitoring systems such as telecare get inserted into people's existing biographies or life stories.

Figure 4.5: Handwritten note from member of telecare citizens' panel

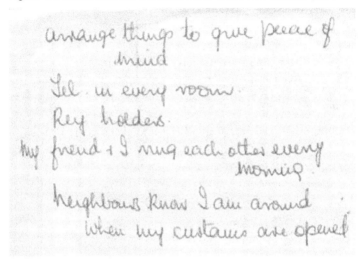

arrange things to give peace of
mind
Tel. in every room.
Key holders.
My friend + I ring each other every
morning.
neighbours know I am around
when my curtains are opened

While welcoming the potential benefits of remote monitoring, participants frequently stressed fears about possible increases in social isolation and loneliness:

> "I think this is one of the things that's coming through over telecare is the fact that people are feeling isolated and because people think they're safe, they're not going round to see them, get in touch with them, or families are thinking 'oh, they've got that, we can …'." (Ellen)

Interestingly, however, it was also recognised that in the most extreme cases of existing isolation, telecare might actually increase social interaction: "I think the thing with human interaction is, some people might actually end up with more interaction through telecare because there are some people who are very isolated who might get to speak to somebody maybe once a week" (Marion).

Others reflected on the ways in which isolated older people might try to use the system to address loneliness:

Eric: "The thing is you'll also get people who will abuse the system, particularly lonely old people … press your button, someone's going to talk to you for five or ten minutes, you know … it's bound to happen."

Jennifer: "I think that's good, I think that's good myself personally."

Eric: "But it tells you what … comfort, it tells you what people want, though, they don't want, they don't really want the automation."

Anne: "They want someone to speak to."

Eric: "They want somebody."

Participants were concerned about what kind of society was being built with the introduction of remote monitoring:

"If it led to an automated society so you got, so the care ended up looking like a milking parlour basically, and those people whose main desire is human touch or a human contact don't get that. And I think most of the people that I'm in contact with want human contact…. The telecare system is ok but if it's not used in conjunction with human contact, then, as I say, it comes down to being unethical and it's purely for money saving, which is, I don't think it's ethical. So I think we do need an education, almost from very young. It's almost a complete change in society to re-educate ourselves to take care. And then the telecare can help us to be taken care of." (Marion)

Automatic alarm sensors led to much debate about intrusiveness and disruption:

Alan: "We've set it off a few times when I've come back
         from the pub at night, and daughter's set it off
         when she's sneaked out for a cigarette, because we
         don't let her smoke in the house, but it doesn't go
         off by itself. Somebody has to set it off. But that
         worries me, for an old person. Having the system
         in the house. Would they understand it? That's the
         other thing. Especially if you've got Alzheimer's,
         it's very hard to explain what it's for, isn't it?"

Penny: "I would never have a mattress sensor because
         I get up and wander now. I've always got up and
         wandered because I don't sleep well. So you know,
         that's something they'd always have to be sure of.
         I mean all my life I've been a poor sleeper and
         so I just get up and walk around and get up and
         go back to bed again, or go and sit in the lounge
         for a bit or whatever. And that's always been my
         pattern of sleep and a mattress sensor would be
         no good for people like me?"

At the disabled people's panel were heard about a politics of
care in which home care itself can impact of people's dignity
and autonomy:

"One of the downsides of having care is that carers
can import their ethos into your home and it does
institutionalise your home in interactions if you get an
insensitive carer. I have had carers who asked 'Does she
take...?' or they are answering endless phone calls to do
with other calls – these are all agendas you don't want
in your home and you don't want to have to fight for
attention in your home. You start to feel that your home
is becoming a public place, a place of work rather than a
place of living." (Mark)

Our qualitative research with older people receiving telecare, with citizens deliberating policy and practice questions around ageing in place, and with carers' groups shows that the most consistently raised concern is not safety and security in the home, but loss of human contact and loneliness (although, of course, these two concerns can be strongly related). Many studies in addition to ours (see Oxlund and Whyte's [2014] review) report that social interaction and face-to-face care is valued most highly by older people as a 'measure' of successful ageing, and that remote care, when it is accepted, is seen either as an extra or as a means to avoid something else – such as ending up in (demonised, but also austerity-hit) residential care. Current telecare systems focus on physical functionality and safety, rather than paying attention to what older people say they value most. However, would the extension of 'smart homes' to include the monitoring of social interactions (as already occurs with Alexa or Google Home) be welcome? Could a metric for social interaction, for example, be generated to go alongside physical functionality in the home? Could devices and platforms be developed to enhance social contacts rather than only monitoring their decline or lack?

Conclusions

Rather than exploring the strong potential of sensor-based monitoring as a form of surveillance within a political economy of ageing (Kenner, 2008) or its normative role in constructions of good or bad ageing (Pickard, 2011), we have focused more closely on the relationship between devices and the body. Biosensing in old age, as exemplified in the increasingly ubiquitous falls detector, appears (and is marketed) as a simple and mundane form of self-care but turns out on closer examination to be anything but simple and to be quite far from self-care. We have seen that for the device to decipher what is and is not a fall has provided the technology companies and so-called users with intractable problems. Too sensitive and the user and monitoring centre are plagued with false alarms; less sensitive and certain falls are not detected. None are actually prevented. Indeed, US computer engineer Tom Doris (2014) describes how the falls detector technology that we have examined here is still in its infancy and the claims often made for these devices can be misleading. The (aged) body-as-sensor aligns poorly with the detector-as-sensor, or, as we argued in the Introduction, the 'inner' sensor misaligns with the 'outer'. A new generation of digital telecare devices is coming with new promises, although Doris warns against future claims to have solved the falls problem in the absence of hard evidence.

However, perhaps some anxiety is managed and a certain peace of mind is afforded simply by the wearing of telecare devices. Certainly, home-care biosensors promise much, and such promise can be alluring and attractive. Families and care organisations find such promise hard to resist given the growing scale of addressing care needs for very old and frail people in the context of demographic change in which ageing is seen as problematic. As in the case of fertility biosensors discussed in Chapter 1, where couples find ovulation monitoring gives them something useful to do while waiting for access to in vitro fertilisation (IVF) interventions, the home monitoring of older people is perhaps a way of queuing or holding 'frail' bodies in a sort of preclinical/pre-residential care zone. Undoubtedly, telecare plays some part in care, some part in the delicate and complex patchwork of care practices, which includes opening and closing the curtains. However, perhaps exchanging messages with a neighbour based on how you move your curtains is more appropriately described as self-tracking than using dys-tracking telecare devices.

Looking back at the biosensors explored in this book, we argue that there is no complete peace of mind, or control, or total solution to whatever the problem is figured to be, but in the case of falls detectors, agency seems more than ever elusive.

While the 'Temperature Egg' does afford a role for the user, we have also seen that data, once inputted, is harvested and manipulated in ways that the so-called user cannot control. With telecare monitoring, data emanates from the device in a way that is beyond the wearer's control, and is only available to certain others who may or may not use it to inform decisions. In the absence of technical solutions to the falling body, traditional forms of care labour (often gendered) are, of course, still required.

In the Introduction, we asked: does the proximity of social care to state or civil society organisations such as social services or charities alter when telecare monitoring platforms connect individuals and social groups differently (family, friends, call centre workers and social workers)? The answer to this question is perhaps not yet, in the sense that the dream (or nightmare) of the at-scale management of older people living at home is yet to be realised – and perhaps also as the more creative hopes that older people living alone might benefit from new forms of connection or sociality through telecare are also largely unrealised. However, it seems likely that biosensing will become part of the formation of aged bodies and the shaping of what counts as care in contemporary contexts with the further development and platformisation of third-generation telecare, as some limited examples show.

Our research in this area, alongside the insights provided by many other kinds of studies, indicates that telecare systems are not (yet) 'good enough', and that they could be so much more creative and flexible. We believe that it is important, as Nafus (2016a: xii) says, to recognise that 'technologies are never a done deal'. She asks: what is to prevent these kinds of biosensors becoming 'the very worst that modernity has to offer'? As mentioned earlier, a biosensor-rich world requires a much more complex notion of where a person's body begins and ends (Nafus, 2016b: 228). Such complexity includes both the 'bio' in the sense of biographical, and the 'bios' in the sense of living, being alive and, by association, having well-being. You may wear an individualising falls detector and hope it communicates with a remote care centre when needed, and/or you may use your curtains to communicate that you are well with your neighbour.

By following the devices in everyday life, illuminating the responses and reactions of, in this case, older people, and bringing forward some perhaps uncomfortable questions, we hope to contribute to a constructive debate about biosensor-based care. By inviting critical thinking about the effects of such systems in daily use and how they are seen to shape new versions of bodies and lives, we can hope to avoid the worst forms of modernity presaged by Nafus.

Conclusion: What Might Biosensing Do?

In 2018, two of us moved to the Australian National University, and in a flurry of new academic encounters, were invited to the inaugural lecture of a Vice-Chancellor's Entrepreneurial Professorial Fellow. Adrian attended and wrote the following field note in **Box C.1**.

Box C.1: Biosensing futures

By Adrian Mackenzie

The auditorium stacks to the back rows, health ministers, local politicians and university dignitaries to the front, and a university audience behind. We sit back to hear about micro-wearables, nano-technology biosensors engineered to 'functionally interface' with the skin. The Entrepreneurial Professorial Fellow's startup will engineer devices that 'gain access to the skin for all manner of signals.' He shows photographs of a small square patch stuck on a forearm like a plaster and a video of an ECG (electrocardiogram) signal, pulsing smoothly. The signal is 'clean' because nano-sized sensor spikes probe interstitial fluids without puncturing cell walls, without needles for blood or vials for urine. In a planned 'biotech skunkworks,' innovation will slalom past pharmaceutical or medical device manufacturers with their fifteen year product pipelines. It will be like Google, he claims, because the biosensor field is moving too fast for the regulatory regimes of medicine. Micro-wearable biosensing, we hear, is more like contemporary cars than clinical observations: 200–2000 continuous signals can be recorded. The data will not only feed into population-level data collection but into profiles of individual variability. In the crowded lobby afterwards, white-aproned waiters pour glasses of local wines and neaten up trays of canapés for the guests. Despite the biotech skunkworks – an interdisciplinary incubator for high-tech – and the vaulting ambitions to change clinical practice in global North and South, the microwearables, should they reach a market, do not figure in the talk or in the chorus of talk in the lobby as elements of a platform. The devices might combine science, engineering and medicine, and they might 'break through the silos between global science, technology and people,' but their alignments with biosensing and its platforms are not mentioned.

More theatrically than most of what we have described in this book, this inaugural lecture was a scene of promise, hope and optimism: that health interventions will not hurt so much; that technological change will be rapid and unhindered by regulation; that universities and corporations will build profitable partnerships; and that biosensing will transform both individual and population health. Biosensing in all its forms, we argue, has strong connections to such promises and the horizon of the 'soon'. Reports about biosensing chime with these promises: X million people are tracking their menstrual cycles; Y million older people are using telecare; and W million have sent their saliva off for genetic testing. Fitbits and Apple Watches are commonplace among the middle-class constituencies that Intel was interested in, and there are countless apps encouraging and helping people to engage with and understand their health-tracking data.

However, it is also possible to unearth counter-narratives, stories of failure, disappointment and limitation: many telecare devices lie on the shelf; people give up quickly on Fitbits; stress biosensing produces inexplicable results; and direct-to-consumer (DTC) genetic test users are more interested in finding obscure cousins than learning about their health. People who use devices to measure stress feel more stressed. Some patients who are given Fitbits to lose weight do less exercise. Monitoring your ovulation does not lead to clarity about fertility, let alone pregnancy.

The yawning gap between these two (tediously familiar) narratives is populated by many interesting stories, not least the emerging body of social-scientific work on biosensing that we have cited throughout, and to which the detailed work of our PhD students and contributing authors – Joann Wilkinson, Mette Kragh-Furbo and Theresa Atkinson – and, indeed, this book belongs. Often, in classical STS (Science and Technology Studies) style, this work highlights the invisible labour that goes on in the gap: Kragh-Furbo describes the spreadsheets designed by people with chronic fatigue used to make connections between 23andMe test results and the effects of nutritional supplements; Wilkinson explores women's collective online efforts to make sense of ferning patterns in saliva; and Atkinson highlights the work of call-centre operators, technical installers, social workers and families in materialising the connections constituting telecare.

In contemporary health care, the unbridged gap between narratives of promise and failure creates a space of wariness, misunderstanding and caution for clinicians and patients. A recent review of relevant literature showed that, like the general practitioner (GP) 'expert witness' at our biosensing citizens' panel, most clinicians have very little interest in, or even awareness of, self-tracking data (West et al, 2017). Except on rare occasions where doctors experimentally prescribe the use of biosensors to support behaviour changes (such as exercise), biosensing data is regarded with great suspicion in clinics. Indeed, patients' interest in self-tracking, West et al (2017: 8) discovered, is often itself viewed as a symptom of ill health (anxiety, obsession, compulsiveness, excessive concern). Presenting data to one's clinician was viewed by some as 'begging for a diagnosis' (West et al, 2017: 8). Clinicians give various reasons for the low value they attribute to biosensing data: the devices used to gather it are not subject to regulation or standards; the data is not standardised; biosensing collects data that is not part of a mainstream medical remit; patients are bad at collecting data and do so haphazardly, so the data may be full of errors or noise; there is too much of it; it often needs a large amount of contextual information to make any sense; there are too many different representations of self-tracking data, which require too much work to comprehend; and the devices and associated apps use language designed for laypeople rather than the language of medical science, among other reasons. West et al (2017: 2) suggest that self-tracked data could, in principle, '"bridge ... the gap" between clinical consultations and letting doctors build an accurate picture of patients over a long period of time', but, as yet does not function in this way.

In this book, we have argued that the gap between the two key biosensing narratives is richly populated by actors, most notably, bodies and platforms. Until we consider bodies in their biopsychosocial fullness and platforms in their equally rich complexity, we will fail to understand what biosensing can and cannot do, and, more importantly, what it might yet do. Platforms are the configured zones where the necessary, multiple meetings that make biosensing possible are enacted. Some of these are high-profile – like Amazon or Google – and some of them are barely visible, embedded in devices and systems. Platforms bring together devices, infrastructures and different social groups, making and breaking connections, mediating and disintermediating relations between things like governments and citizens, corporations and customers, institutions and publics. Articulating and analysing the platforms means exploring how things are arranged to make some kinds of biosensing possible and asking what might need to be gathered together to make new kinds. Such work allows us to see the power relations that platforms typically cover over.

This book has also argued that we need to centre discussion on bodies and '*bio*' in all its senses. Building on several decades of scholarship on the body in feminist, queer and poststructuralist theory, as well as STS, medical sociology, sociology, disability studies and cultural and media studies, we understand bodies to be biopsychosocial. Indeed, we have suggested here that, even at their worst, biosensing practices can help us to articulate the complex intra-actions (Barad, 2007) of biological, psychological and social forces in lived experience. In the preceding chapters, we have discussed issues pertaining to patterns of hormonal changes, gene expression, menstrual flows and falling bodies.

We have emphasised the significance of felt (mentally processed) stress, of loneliness and of desire for familial and other new forms of human connection. Moving across the life course – from childhood, through the so-called 'reproductive years' and into older age – we have argued that biosensing is producing new understandings of what constitutes a (healthy) life, and highlighted the significance of geographical, historical and social location in this. Biosensing gunshot-related stress in urban Chicago is a very different practice to self-tracking heart rate in Finland. Using DTC genetic tests to find out about one's ancestors and relatives in Africa as a young black American wanting to trace vectors of pride and survival has a particular valence and power. Buying a smart house system like Alexa for the excitement and possible benefits of having the latest techno kit has little resonance with being an older person living in a deprived part of North England prescribed with a falls monitor and less-than-satisfactory face-to-face care. To put it bluntly, what bodies do, how they are lived and understood, and in what social, cultural and economic circumstances they exist really matter in understanding biosensing.

West et al (2017) found that biosensing data is currently of little relevance to clinical encounters, despite all the promise and hype decorating the scene. We do not – and may never – have the right platforms to stage helpful meetings between people who self-track, biosensing devices, apps and systems, the data they create, display and analyse, and doctors and their spaces of clinical assessment, observation and intervention. Biosensing may be about health for many people but it, as yet, has little to do with biomedicine.

Energetic debate is currently taking place in the social sciences around whether biosensing is changing human health. In many ways, as we have discussed, the scene seems full of failure and disappointment: bodies do not change much in response to being tracked. But there are also moments of intrigue and surprise in biosensing that may be life-changing: becoming convinced that you do ovulate might change your experience of infertility; noting that picking up your child from childcare tracks with a spike in physiological stress may help you rethink your practices; you might live better with a chronic condition such as Chronic Fatigue Syndrome by experimenting with foods attuned to different DNA methylation patterns; and allowing an older person with dementia to 'wander' because they are wearing a tracking device might contribute to everyone's well-being (EFORTT Researchers, 2011). Biosensing, in our view, has the potential to change human bodies and lives in, as yet, barely imagined ways. To track and understand these changes – and to work towards designing devices and systems that will promote health, equality and freedom – we must pay serious attention to both the technologies and platforms constituting 'sensing' and to the 'bio' in their equally rich complexities.

Health biosensing policy and practice

What conclusions can we draw for those working in relevant areas of policy and practice (whether technology design, clinical medicine, health activism or other fields)? Most importantly, we want to suggest that all such work should, like future research, pay attention to platforms and bodies when addressing health biosensing. Promissory narratives focused on devices – that 'soon' things will be better, that a 'computer-savvy' generation will manage technology better and that devices will be smaller, faster and simpler to use – are easy stories to tell. The risks of such stories are twofold: first, they may never come true; and, second, they may cause harm either by distracting us from what is already going on, or by limiting our imaginings of alternative futures. Turning down the volume on promissory announcements leaves space to listen to diverse experiences and to imagine and explore what people (that is, citizens, not only stakeholders, but anyone who is interested) might want biosensing to be, and what they are afraid it might do. Citizens' panels, ethnographic research, critical textual analysis and forms of experimental participatory design generate much-needed alternative narratives for policy and design, opening up questions and concerns, pointing to problematic inheritances, and possibly limiting entanglements. Policymakers, industry bodies and corporations, and activists interested in health biosensing could do well to devote time and resources, as did Intel Labs, to listening to and engaging with 'the word on the street', as filtered through social science. People of all ages and backgrounds are thinking about, using and/or encountering health biosensing – living data – and they have much to say about its liveliness. We hope that this book will be part of these ongoing conversations.

Appendix

Scenario: the Browns from Preston: an 'ordinary family'

Theresa, grandmother died at 75 with Alzheimer's disease

John, 65, Theresa's son, becoming forgetful

Cath, 60, John's wife, concerned about her husband and son

Ben, 32, John and Cath's son, single, uses genetic testing kit from 23andMe, found to have an 'increased risk of Alzheimer's disease'

Louise, 36, John and Cath's daughter, married, infertility issues, uses ovulation microscope

Yusef, 30, Louise's husband, infertility issues

Act 1: making sense of genetic data

Ben is a single man with a good job working in a small engineering company. He likes computers and his smartphone and enjoys downloading films and surfing the web. One of his recent favourite websites is called 23andMe. This is a company based in the US that sells genetic testing kits directly to the public. A friend at work had read about 23andMe in the magazine *Wired* and mentioned it over lunch one day. He had been quite excited about it.

Three months ago, Ben sent off for a genetic testing kit from 23andMe's website, and when it arrived, he followed the instructions as pictured in the package. He registered the kit on the website and filled in the online form with his name, gender and date of birth. It also asked him if he wanted to take online surveys and be part of 23andMe's research studies. He read through the consent document and ticked the box: 'Yes, I'd like to participate in making new genetic discoveries with 23andMe Research'. He took out the small 'spittoon' that came with the box, spat into the tube and sealed it according to the instructions. His favourite part of the kit was the biohazard logo on the plastic bag that came with the tube.

Five weeks later, he got an email from 23andMe saying that his results were ready and that they would tell him all about his 'personal genome', about the patterns in his DNA and what they mean for his health, the way his body works, and even his family history running back centuries. Ben is healthy, and did not expect any bad news. His main reason for having the test was curiosity. He read through his results, which said all kinds of things, such as that he was unlikely to be a sprinter and that his earwax type was wet. His risk of deep vein thrombosis was also lower than average. But there was one thing that was a bit alarming in his test results. Ben carries one copy of something called the ApoE4 allele, which gives him an above normal risk of getting Alzheimer's disease.

Now, his grandmother, Theresa, had died with Alzheimer's disease at the age of 75. Ben had never thought much about that until now. Come to think of it, his mother, Cath, had recently been saying that his father, John, was having problems remembering lots of small things day to day. He would forget names and misplace things. Ben kept thinking about his 23andMe results, and the thought that he might get Alzheimer's stuck in his mind. He started spending quite a lot of time on the 23andMe website and its community forum reading postings about other people's test results. Many of them had taken their results to their doctors, and some were taking nutritional supplements to lower their risk of getting Alzheimer's disease.

There was a lot of discussion about the family history of the condition, and quite a lot of references to and talk about medical and scientific papers that people had read. Ben started to search for scientific papers and read several dozen that he found on the web but found them pretty confusing. Some reported a 'twofold increased risk with the ApoE4 allele', but some of the papers reported a threefold lifetime risk. He was not sure how to make sense of all the information and his own test results, so he made an appointment to see his GP. But the visit was not a success, the doctor did not seem to know much about recent research on the genetics of Alzheimer's and could not make sense of the 23andMe results. Although his GP reminded him that the information only suggested a risk, Ben still felt worried.

A few days after, he brought up the test results when talking with his mother. Her immediate reaction was concern. She also thought that Ben's father should take the test, but John was not interested. He would face it when and if the time came. Ben felt differently. He wanted to know more about what he could do to prevent Alzheimer's, and since his GP was not much help, he went back onto 23andMe's website to look for answers.

Act 2: making sense of fertility monitoring

Ben's sister, Louise, aged 36, was having troubles of her own. Louise was a full-time pre-school teacher and really wanted to have children. Five years ago, she married Yusef, aged 30, who she had met on holiday in Turkey. The couple had been trying to start a family for about a year now and were becoming concerned that there might be some deeper, underlying medical issues that might be affecting their fertility. About two months ago, Louise came across an article in a magazine about conception and pregnancy that described a few ways in which women are monitoring ovulation in order to help them conceive. Louise knew vaguely that there was a more fertile time of the month, but she did not know much about ovulation or when those fertile times might be. According to the article, if Louise knew when she ovulated, she and Yusef would have a much better chance of conceiving. One of the technologies that the article recommended was the ovulation microscope. It was a small device that looked like a lipstick and had a compact microscopic lens inside. It seemed relatively straightforward to use, and at only £12.99, was pretty affordable. Louise decided that she would try and buy it at Boots but could not find it, and the shop assistants had not heard of it either.

Browsing online, she found she could buy it directly from the manufacturer's website; they even had other products, such as for testing the quality of sperm or for the menopause. When it arrived, she found the device to be much smaller and more compact than she had imagined; it looked like a lipstick but, somehow, she had imagined it to be more scientific or technical. She examined it, reading the instructions and studying the black-and-white photos of ovulation patterns. Feeling excited, she placed it on her bedside table ready for the morning. According to the instructions, she had to use the device before eating or drinking anything, not even a glass of water, and also before brushing her teeth as this would affect the saliva and make it more difficult to see the ovulation patterns on the lens. When morning came, just seconds after waking up, Louise opened the microscope and unscrewed the lens. She placed a small amount of saliva onto the clean glass. She waited nervously for several minutes and then examined the patterns that had formed on the lens, but she could not see anything; no shapes, no patterns, just a blank yellow space. According to the instruction sheet this meant that she was not fertile on that day. She was somewhat disappointed but thought that perhaps she was expecting too much on her first day! She made a note of the data on her smartphone – she had downloaded an app that made it easier for her to keep a record of her fertile and non-fertile days, as well as other bits of information, such as menstruation dates, aches and pains, moods, and anything else that might indicate ovulation or, perhaps even one day, pregnancy. After eight days, she gradually began to see patterns emerge; they were like crystals in the shape of ferns. According to the instructions, this meant that she was ovulating. She began to feel excited about this. Even though ovulation was something that happened every month, this time it was different, she could see it happening; somehow, she was more involved in the process and more in tune with her body. It also made her feel that she was getting closer to what she really wanted, a child. She told Yusef about it but he was less enthusiastic, "Let's just keep trying and see how it goes" he always said, which annoyed her. They both wanted children, but she seemed to want it more, perhaps this was because he was younger; he had more time.

She continued to use the ovulation microscope over several days and months, storing the data in her smartphone. She could now easily recognise the days when she was ovulating, yet there was no sign of pregnancy. Why? She had felt so optimistic when she bought the microscope; now disappointment was setting in. She looked at some of the pregnancy forums on the Internet where women discussed using the microscope and shared their experiences. She found that some were uploading pictures of their ovulating patterns and discussing what the images meant. Although some women had become pregnant while using the microscope, others had not and were looking for alternatives.

Ten months later, Louise was using the microscope less and less. She was able to feel when ovulation took place, the microscope had helped her with that, but she was still not pregnant. She knew that she would have to go and see her GP soon to talk about other options. She was anxious about this and about what her GP might say. She had chatted to other women on online forums and many of these had chosen to go down the IVF path. What other path was there actually? The prospect of infertility treatment and all that came with it was frightening.

Some of the other women on the forum had recommended the 'Duo-Fertility Monitor' as the last step before IVF. This was another fertility monitor but one that was supposedly much more sophisticated, although some women described it as a 'fancy, expensive thermometer'. At £500, it was certainly expensive, but then again, IVF could end up costing a lot more. Louise looked this device up on the Internet and read the reviews of women users. There were two parts to it; one was a coin like piece that had to be worn under the arm and the other was an egg-shaped monitor that had lots of symbols on it. The coin piece took 20,000 temperature readings a day, which were then sent to the egg-shaped monitor. It was also possible to add in your own data – it was a bit like a diary. All of this data would then be uploaded onto your computer and sent to the Duo Fertility Centre. Fertility specialists would look through the data and identify signs of ovulation or any problems with fertility. To Louise, this all sounded really positive. She had already made contact with one of the fertility experts and he seemed helpful, taking time to respond to her questions. If she were to buy the Duo Fertility monitor, it would also mean that she would be able to hold off on any (medical) fertility treatment for the time being. After ten months of trying and failing, was £500 really all that much? She did not think so but was sure that Yusef would not see it that way. Moreover, he should probably also have his sperm tested. Louise was worried about what lay ahead, nothing was clear-cut and there was a lot at stake.

References

23andMe (2018a) 23andMe. Available at: www.23andme.com (accessed 1 March 2018).

23andMe (2018b) 23andMe API. Available at: https://api.23andme.com/ (accessed 28 February 2018).

23andMe (2018c) Explore 23andMe's scientific discoveries UK. Available at: www.23andme.com/en-gb/publications/ (accessed 28 February 2018).

23andMe (2018d) Research. 23andMe UK. Available at: www.23andme.com/en-gb/research/ (accessed 28 February 2018).

23andMe (2018e) Share and Compare. 23andMe. Available at: https://you.23andme.com/tools/share/ (accessed 27 February 2018).

23andMe (2018f) The science behind 23andMe UK. Available at: www.23andme.com/en-gb/genetic-science/ (accessed 28 February 2018).

Akrich, M. (1992) The de-scription of technical objects. In: Bijker, W.E. and Law, J. (eds) *Shaping technology/building society. Studies in sociotechnical change*. Cambridge, MA, and London: MIT Press.

Almeling, R. (2007) Selling genes, selling gender: egg agencies, sperm banks, and the medical market in genetic material. *American Sociological Review* 72(3): 319–40.

Apple Inc (2018) Use the Breathe app. Apple Support. Available at: https://support.apple.com/en-au/HT206999 (accessed 25 November 2018).

Arcana, R. and Indira, S. (2013). Soldier monitoring and health indication system. *International Journal of Science and Research* 4(5): 1150–2.

Atkinson, T. (2019) *Enacting telecare at scale: a study of sociomaterial practices*. Unpublished PhD thesis. Lancaster: Lancaster University.

Barad, K. (2007) *Meeting the universe halfway: Quantum physics and the entanglement of matter and meaning*. Durham, NC: Duke University Press.

Barlyn, S. (2018) Strap on the Fitbit: John Hancock to sell only interactive life insurance. *Reuters*. 19 September. Available at: https://uk.reuters.com/article/us-manulife-financi-john-hancock-lifeins/strap-on-the-fitbit-john-hancock-to-sell-only-interactive-life-insurance-idUKKCN1LZ1WL

Bell, J. (2018) Tips for using Clue when you're trans. 28 March. Available at: https://helloclue.com/articles/cycle-a-z/tips-for-using-clue-when-you%27re-trans (accessed 14 October 2018).

Bennett, J. (2009) *Vibrant matter: A political ecology of things*. Durham, NC: Duke University Press Books.

Bergman, K., Rubio, R.J., Green, R.-J. and Padrón, E. (2010) Gay men who become fathers via surrogacy: the transition to parenthood. *Journal of GLBT Family Studies* 6(2): 111–41.

Bijker, W.E. and Law, J. (eds) (1994) *Shaping technology/building society: Studies in sociotechnical change* (new edn). Cambridge, MA: MIT Press.

Biodesk (2018) Menopause symptoms checklist. 28 September. Available at: https://biodesk.wordpress.com/ (accessed 9 November 2018).

BioWink GmbH (2018) Clue – period & health tracker. *App Store Preview*. Available at: https://itunes.apple.com/app/id657189652?mt=8 (accessed 14 October 2018).

Bloss, C.S., Ornowski, L., Silver, E., Cargill, M., Vanier, V., Schork, N.J. and Topol, E.J. (2010) Consumer perceptions of direct-to-consumer personalized genomic risk assessments. *Genetics in Medicine* 12(9): 556–66.

Böhlen, M. 2016. Field notes in contamination studies. In: Nafus, D. (ed) *Quantified: Biosensing technologies in everyday life* (1st edn). Cambridge, MA: MIT Press, pp 169-88.

Bradley, C. (2017) *Revealing the inner world of traumatised children and young people: An attachment-informed model for assessing emotional needs and treatment*. London: Jessica Kingsley Publishers.

Brigham, K. (2018) Women are using fertility apps as contraception, but experts are skeptical. 9 June. Available at: www.cnbc.com/2018/06/08/women-are-using-fertility-apps-as-contraception-but-experts-are-skeptical.html (accessed 24 November 2018).

Building Better Healthcare (2013) Tunstall launches fall detection alarm. Available at: www.buildingbetterhealthcare.co.uk/news/article_page/Tunstall_launches_fall_detection_alarm/88127 (accessed 29 November 2018).

Buniello A., MacArthur J.A.L., Cerezo M., Harris L.W., Hayhurst J., Malangone C., McMahon A., Morales J., Mountjoy E., Sollis E., Suveges D., Vrousgou O., Whetzel P.L., Amode R., Guillen J.A., Riat H.S., Trevanion S.J., Hall P., Junkins H., Flicek P., Burdett T., Hindorff L.A., Cunningham F. and Parkinson H. (2019) The NHGRI-EBI GWAS Catalog of published genome-wide association studies, targeted arrays and summary statistics 2019. *Nucleic Acids Research*, 47: D1005-D1012.

Bury, M. (1982) Chronic illness as biographical disruption. *Sociology of Health & Illness* 4(2): 167–82.

Caddy, B. (2018) Stress tracking tech: heart rate monitoring and guided breathing devices. *Wareable*, 22 June. Available at: www.wareable.com/wearable-tech/stress-beating-tech-to-keep-you-sane (accessed 7 November 2018).

Campbell, J. and Ehlert, U. (2012) Acute psychosocial stress: does the emotional stress response correspond with physiological responses? *Psychoneuroendocrinology* 37(8): 1111–34.

Canguilhem, G. (1989) *On the normal and the pathological* (trans Fawcett, C.R.). Cambridge, MA: Zone Books.

Cannon, W. (1963) *Wisdom of the body* (revised and enlarged edn). New York, NY: W.W. Norton & Company.

CB Insights (2017) The femtech market map. Available at: https://www.cbinsights.com/research/report/womens-health-technology-transforming/ (accessed 3 May 2018).

Charara, S. (2015) Muse review: the brain sensing headband that knows you're stressed. *Wareable*, 21 April. Available at: www.wareable.com/wearable-tech/muse-brain-sensing-headband-review-938 (accessed 7 November 2018).

Charara, S. (2016) Bellabeat Leaf Urban review. *Wareable*, 24 October. Available at: www.wareable.com/health-and-wellbeing/bellabeat-leaf-urban-review (accessed 7 November 2018).

Chaudhuri, S. (2018) Fertility apps are multiplying. But are they reliable? *Wall Street Journal*, 24 May. Available at: https://www.wsj.com/articles/fertility-apps-are-multiplying-but-are-they-reliable-1527182930

Chen, B.X. (2018) Apple Watch series 4 review: a big step for wearable gadgets. *The New York Times*, 21 September. Available at: https://www.nytimes.com/2018/09/19/technology/personaltech/apple-watch-series-4-review-health.html

Ciorap, R.G. (2017) Vital signs monitoring during combat actions. Paper presented at the international scientific conference 'Strategies XXI', Bucharest, "Carol I" National Defence University.

Clarke, A.E., Mamo, L., Fosket, J.R., Fishman, J.R. and Shim, J.K. (eds) (2010) *Biomedicalization: Technoscience, health, and illness in the U.S.* Durham, NC: Duke University Press.

Clue (2018) The science of your cycle: evidence-based app design. Available at: https://helloclue.com/articles/about-clue/science-your-cycle-evidence-based-app-design (accessed 17 October 2018).

Collins, S. (2018) Let's talk about periods. 8 March. Available at: www.youtube.com/watch?v=4eVZj-OLZBM (accessed 10 November 2018).

Connell-Tatum, E. (1981) Ovulation method of natural family planning. *Fertility and Sterility* 36(5): 551–2.

Convery, I., Mort, M., Baxter, J. and Bailey, C. (2008) *Animal Disease and Human Trauma: Emotional Geographies of Disaster.* Basingstoke: Palgrave Macmillan.

Cook, J. (2016) German period tracking app Clue has over 2.5 million active users – but it's still not sure how it's going to make money. *Business Insider Australia*, 9 January. Available at: www.businessinsider.com.au/interview-with-clue-ceo-ida-tin-period-tracking-app-apple-2016-1?r=US&IR=T (accessed 2 March 2018).

Crawford, K., Lingel, J. and Karppi, T. (2015) Our metrics, ourselves: a hundred years of self-tracking from the weight scale to the wrist wearable device. *European Journal of Cultural Studies* 18(4/5): 479–96.

Davies, W. (2015) *The happiness industry: How the government and big business sold us well-being.* London: Verso.

DNA.LAND (2018) Homepage. Available at: https://dna.land/ (accessed 2 March 2018).

Donovan, S. (2013) *No matter what: An adoptive family's story of hope, love and healing*. London and Philadelphia, PA: Jessica Kingsley Publishers.

Doris, T. (2014) Accelerometers, false positives/negatives and fall detection. *Telehealth & Telecare Aware*. Available at: http://telecareaware.com/accelerometers-false-positivesnegatives-and-fall-detection/ (accessed 10 November 2018).

Dreaper, J. (2016) Women warned about booming market in period tracker apps. *BBC News*. 11 August. Available at: www.bbc.com/news/health-37013217 (accessed 1 February 2018).

Druet, A. (2018) Scientific research at Clue. How tracking your cycle advances female health. 27 March. Available at: https://helloclue.com/articles/about-clue/scientific-research-at-clue (accessed 12 June 2018).

EFORTT (Ethical Frameworks for Telecare Technologies) (2008) Available at: www.lancaster.ac.uk/efortt/

EFORTT Researchers (2011) Final Report of Ethical Frameworks for Telecare Technologies for older people at home. EU FP7 Project 217787. Available at: www.lancaster.ac.uk/efortt/ (accessed 29 November 2018).

Ehm, M.G., Aponte, J.L., Chiano, M.N., Yerges-Armstrong, L.M., Johnson, T., Barker, J.N., Cook, S.F., Gupta, A., Hinds, D.A., Li, L., Nelson, M.R., Simpson, M.A., Tian, C., McCarthy, L.C., Rajpal, D.K. and Waterworth, D.M. (2017) Phenome-wide association study using research participants' self-reported data provides insight into the Th17 and IL-17 pathway. *PLOS ONE* 12(11): e0186405.

Empatica Inc (2018) Embrace seizure detection – manage epilepsy – SUDEP. *Empatica*. Available at: www.empatica.com/embrace (accessed 7 November 2018).

Epstein, D.A., Lee, N.B., Kang, J.H., Agapie, E., Schroeder, J., Pina, L.R., Fogarty, J., Kientz, J.A. and Munson, S.A. (2017) Examining menstrual tracking to inform the design of personal informatics tools. In: *Proceedings of the SIGCHI conference on human factors in computing systems. CHI Conference*, pp 6876–88.

EU (European Union) (2016) EUR-Lex – 32016R0679 – EN – EUR-Lex. Available at: https://eur-lex.europa.eu/eli/reg/2016/679/oj (accessed 19 October 2018).

Faulkner, A. (2009) *Medical technology into healthcare and society: A sociology of devices, innovation and governance*. Basingstoke: Palgrave Macmillan.

Financial Review (2015) Why your boss wants you to wear biosensing devices. *Financial Review*, 12 August. Available at: www.afr.com/leadership/innovation/why-your-boss-wants-you-to-wear-biosensing-devices-20150812-gixkfz (accessed 30 November 2018).

Fiore-Gartland, B. and Neff, G. (2016) Disruption and the political economy of biosensor data. In: Nafus, D. (ed) *Quantified: Biosensing technologies in everyday life*. Cambridge, MA, and London: MIT Press, pp 10–22.

Fitabase (2018) Fitabase – research device data and analytics. Available at: www.fitabase.com/ (accessed 15 October 2018).

Fitbit (2018) What should I know about the Relax app on my Fitbit device? *Fitbit Help*. Available at: https://help.fitbit.com/articles/en_US/Help_article/2077 (accessed 7 November 2018).

Fleming, J. and Brayne, C. (2008) Inability to get up after falling, subsequent time on floor, and summoning help: prospective cohort study in people over 90. *BMJ* 337: a2227.

Flemings, M., Pak, R., Kazmi, S. and Shaer, O. (2018) Crimson wave: shedding light on menstrual health. *TEI '18 Proceedings of the Twelfth International Conference on Tangible, Embedded, and Embodied Interaction*. Stockholm, Sweden.

Forth (2018a) Cortisol test kit – cortisol blood test at home – private level check. *Forth*. Available at: www.forthwithlife.co.uk/cortisol/ (accessed 29 November 2018).

Forth (2018b) General wellbeing tests. *Forth*. Available at: www.forthwithlife.co.uk/wellbeing/ (accessed 7 November 2018).

Forth (2018c) Baseline plus – full, advanced blood tests for health screening. *Forth*. Available at:www.forthwithlife.co.uk/baseline-plus/ (accessed 7 November 2018).

Foucault, M. (1988) *The history of sexuality: The use of pleasure*. New York, NY: Vintage Books.

Foucault, M. (1990) *History of sexuality. Vol.1: An introduction*. Harmondsworth: Penguin.

Fox, J. (2017) How tech is transforming fertility tracking – for lads and ladies. *ABC News*, 19 February. Available at: www.abc.net.au/news/2017-02-19/technology-is-transforming-fertility-men-and-women/8268046 (accessed 10 November 2018).

Franklin, S. (1997) *Embodied progress: A cultural account of assisted conception* (1st edn). London and New York, NY: Routledge.

Franklin, S. (2013) *Biological relatives: IVF, stem cells, and the future of kinship*. Durham, NC: Duke University Press.

Franklin, S. and Roberts, C. (2006) *Born and made: An ethnography of pre-implantation genetic diagnosis*. Princeton, NJ, and Oxford: Princeton University Press.

GenesForGood (2018) Genes for Good. Available at: https://genesforgood.sph.umich.edu/ (accessed 2 March 2018).

Genos (2018) Genos – own your DNA. Available at: https://genos.co (accessed 2 March 2018).

Greenfield, D. (2016) Deep data: notes on the n of 1. In: Nafus, D. (ed) *Quantified: Biosensing technologies in everyday life*. Cambridge, MA, and London: MIT Press, pp 123–67.

Gregory, J. and Bowker, G.C. (2016) The data citizen, the quantified self, and personal genomics. In: Nafus, D. (ed) *Quantified: Biosensing technologies in everyday life*. Cambridge, MA, and London: MIT Press, pp 211–22.

Haraway, D.J. (1997) *Modest_Witness@Second_Millennium.FemaleMan_Meets_OncoMouse: Feminism and technoscience*. New York, NY, and London: Routledge.

Harris, A., Kelly, S. and Wyatt, S. (2016) *CyberGenetics: Health genetics and new media*. London and New York, NY: Routledge, Taylor & Francis Group.

Hauskeller, C. (2011) Direct to consumer genetic testing. *BMJ (Clinical Research Edn)* 342: d2317.

Helmond, A. (2015) The platformization of the web: making web data platform ready. *Social Media + Society* 1(2): 1–11.

Henderson, C., Knapp, M., Fernández, J.-L., Beecham, J., Hirani, S.P., Beynon, M., Cartwright, M., Rixon, L., Doll, H., Bower, P., Steventon, A., Rogers, A., Fitzpatrick, R., Barlow, J., Bardsley, M. and Newman, S.P. (2014) Cost-effectiveness of telecare for people with social care needs: the Whole Systems Demonstrator cluster randomised trial. *Age and Ageing* 43(6): 794–800.

Hercher, L. (2018) Opinion – 23andMe said he would lose his mind. Ancestry said the opposite. Which was right? *The New York Times*, 15 September. Available at: https://www.nytimes.com/2018/09/15/opinion/sunday/23andme-ancestry-alzheimers-genetic-testing.html

Hesse, B.W., Nelson, D.E., Kreps, G.L., Croyle, R.T., Neeraj, A.K., Rimer, B.K. and Kastomayatjula, V. (2005) Trust and sources of health information: the impact of the Internet and its implications for health care providers: findings from the first Health Information National Trends Survey. *Archives of Internal Medicine* 165(December): 2618–24.

Homewood, S. (2018) Ambient cycle. *Sarah Homewood Interaction Design*. Available at: http://sarahhomewood.com/AmbientCycle.html

Hoyt, R.W., Reifman, J., Coster, T.S. and Buller, M.J. (2002) Combat medical informatics: present and future. *Proceedings of the AMIA Symposium*: 335–9.

Hughes, D.A. (1998) *Building the bonds of attachment: Awakening love in deeply troubled children.* Lanham, MD: Rowman & Littlefield.

Hughes, D.A. and Baylin, J. (2012) *Brain-based parenting: The neuroscience of caregiving for healthy attachment.* New York and London: W.W. Norton & Company.

Husain, I. and Spence, D. (2015) Can healthy people benefit from health apps? *BMJ* 350: h1887.

Igual, R., Medrano, C. and Plaza, I. (2013) Challenges, issues and trends in fall detection systems. *BioMedical Engineering OnLine* 12(1): 66.

Infinome (2018) Fight obesity by sharing your data and helping science. Available at: https://infino.me/welcome (accessed 24 September 2018).

Inhorn, M. and Patrizio, P. (2015) Infertility around the globe: new thinking on gender, reproductive technologies and global movements in the 21st century. *Human Reproduction Update* 21(4): 411–26.

Jackson, M. (2013) *The age of stress: Science and the search for stability*. Oxford: Oxford University Press.

James, W. (1976) *Essays in radical empiricism* (vol 3). Cambridge, MA: Harvard University Press.

Jameson, F. (1991) *Postmodernism, or, the cultural logic of late capitalism*. Durham, NC: Duke University Press.

John, N.A. (2013) Sharing and Web 2.0: the emergence of a keyword. *New Media & Society* 15(2): 167–82.

Kashefi, E. and Mort, M. (2004) Grounded citizens' juries: a tool for health activism? *Health Expectations: An International Journal of Public Participation in Health Care and Health Policy* 7(4): 290–302.

Katz, S. and Marshall, B.L. (2018) Tracked and fit: FitBits, brain games, and the quantified aging body. *Journal of Aging Studies* 45: 63–8.

Keating, P. and Cambrosio, A. (2003) *Biomedical platforms: Realigning the normal and the pathological in late-twentieth-century medicine*. Cambridge, MA: MIT Press.

Keller, E.F. (2001) *The century of the gene*. Cambridge, MA, London: Harvard University Press.

Keller, E.F. (2005) The century beyond the gene. *Journal of Biosciences* 30(1): 3–10.

Kenner, A.M. (2008) Securing the elderly body: dementia, surveillance, and the politics of 'aging in place'. *Surveillance & Society* 5(3): 252-69.

Kennett, D. (2018) Personal genetic testing and the implications for the donor conception community. *Bionews*, 26 February. Available at: www.bionews.org.uk/page_934804.asp (accessed 27 February 2018).

Khan, M., Khan, A.R., Shin, J.-H. and Park, S.-Y. (2016) A liquid-crystal-based DNA biosensor for pathogen detection. *Scientific Reports* 6: 22676.

Kimura, S. and Inose, K. (forthcoming) Has ANT been helpful for public anthropology after the 3.11 disaster in Japan? In: Blok, A., Farias, I. and Roberts, C. (eds) *The Routledge companion to actor network theory: A companion*. London: Routledge.

Kragh-Furbo, M., Mackenzie, A., Mort, M. and Roberts, C. (2016) Do biosensors biomedicalize? Sites of negotiation in DNA-based biosensing data practices. In: Nafus, D. (ed) *Quantified: Biosensing technologies in everyday life*. Cambridge and Malden, MA: MIT Press, pp 5-26.

Kragh-Furbo, M., Wilkinson, J., Mort, M., Roberts, C. and Mackenzie, A. (2017) Biosensing networks: sense making in consumer genomics and ovulation tracking. In: Farrington, C. and Lynch, R. (eds) *Personal medical devices: New conceptual approaches in the social sciences and humanities*. Basingstoke: Palgrave-Macmillan, pp 47–70.

Laidler, S. (2017) What is heart rate variability testing and how can you use it to get healthier? *The Telegraph*, 31 January. Available at: www.telegraph.co.uk/men/thinking-man/heart-rate-variability-testing-can-use-get-healthier/ (accessed 7 November 2018).

Latour, B. (1992) Where are the missing masses? The sociology of a few mundane artifacts. In: Bijker, W.E. and Law, J. (eds) *Shaping technology/building society: Studies in sociotechnical change*. Cambridge and Malden, MA: MIT Press, pp 225–58.

Lederbogen, F., Kirsch, P., Haddad, L., Streit, F., Tost, H., Schuch, P., Wüst, S., Pruessner, J.C., Rietschel, M., Deuschle, M. and Meyer-Lindenberg, A. (2011) City living and urban upbringing affect neural social stress processing in humans. *Nature* 474(7352): 498–501.

Leibenger, D., Möllers, F., Petrlic, A., Petrlic, R. and Sorge, C. (2016) Privacy challenges in the quantified self movement – an EU perspective. *Proceedings on Privacy Enhancing Technologies* 4: 315–34.

Levy, K.E.C. (2015) Intimate surveillance. *Idaho Law Review* 51: 679–711.

Lippman, H. (2013). How apps are changing family medicine. *Journal of Family Practice* 62(7): 362–68.

Living Data Research Group (2013) Our bodies our data. Available at: https://livingdata.wordpress.com/our-bodies-our-data/ (accessed 9 November 2018).

Looker, T. and Gregson, O. (2003 [1997]) *Managing stress.* London: Teach Yourself Books.

Lupton, D. (2014) The commodification of patient opinion: the digital patient experience economy in the age of big data. *Sociology of Health & Illness* 36(6): 856–69.

Lupton, D. (2015) Quantified sex: a critical analysis of sexual and reproductive self-tracking using apps. *Culture, Health & Sexuality* 17(4): 440–53.

Lynch, B. (2019) StrateGene: genetic report by Dr Ben Lynch. Available at: http://go.strategene.org/genetic-analysis (accessed 9th May).

Mackenzie, A. (2017) *Machine learners: Archaeology of a data practice.* Cambridge, MA: MIT Press.

Mackenzie, A. (2018) From API to AI: platforms and their opacities. *Information, Communication & Society*, doi: 10.1080/1369118X.2018.1476569.

Mackenzie, A. and Roberts, C. (2017) Adopting neuroscience: parenting and affective indeterminacy. *Body & Society* 23(3): 130–55.

Marina, S., Marina, D., Marina, F., Fosas, N., Galiana, N. and Jové, I. (2010) Sharing motherhood: biological lesbian co-mothers, a new IVF indication. *Human Reproduction* 25(4): 938–41.

Marshall, B.L. and Katz, S. (2016) How old am I? *Digital Culture & Society* 2(1): 145–52.

Maslakovic, M. (2017) Vitali: stay balanced and stress-free with this stylish bra. *Gadgets & Wearables*, 12 April. Available at: https://gadgetsandwearables.com/2017/04/12/vitali-bra/ (accessed 7 November 2018).

Matthews-King, A. (2018) Social care crisis: over-85s needing 24 hour care set to double by 2035, major study shows. *The Independent*, 30 August. Available at: www.independent.co.uk/news/health/elderly-care-double-retirement-pension-age-full-time-care-24-hour-lancet-newcastle-a8514881.html (accessed 29 November 2018).

McCarthy, M. (2013) Experts warn on data security in health and fitness apps. *British Medical Journal* 347: f5600.

McCartney, P.R. (2016) The electronic health record and nursing practice. *The American Journal of Maternal/Child Nursing* 41(2): 126.

McNeil, M. (2007) *Feminist cultural studies of science and technology*. London: Routledge.

Mendenhall, R., Lleras, C., McKee, M., Srinivasan, S., Browne, M., Sergeevna Mainzer, L., Gilleade, K. and Wang, S. (2018) *Using wearable sensors and affective diaries to document how violence affects public life and public health*. Lleras Lab – University of Illinois at Urbana-Champaign. Available at: https://publish.illinois.edu/lleraslab/projects/projectsusing-wearable-sensors-and-affective-diaries-to-document-how-violence-affects-public-life-and-public-health/

Milligan, C., Roberts, C. and Mort, M. (2011) Telecare and older people: who cares where? *Social Science & Medicine* 72(3): 347–54.

Moglia, M.L., Nguyen, H.V., Chyjek, K., Chen, K.T. and Castaño, P.M. (2016) Evaluation of smartphone menstrual cycle tracking applications using an adapted applications scoring system. *Obstetrics & Gynecology* 127(6): 1153.

Montgomery, R.R. and Anderson, Y.L. (2016) *Battlefield medical network: biosensors in a tactical environment*. Master's thesis, Naval Postgraduate School, Monterey, California. Available at: https://core.ac.uk/download/pdf/36740638.pdf

Mort, M., Finch, T. and May, C. (2009) Making and unmaking telepatients: identity and governance in new health technologies. *Science, Technology, & Human Values* 34(1): 9–33.

Mort, M., Roberts, C. and Callén, B. (2013) Ageing with telecare: care or coercion in austerity? *Sociology of Health & Illness* 35(6): 799–812.

Mort, M., Roberts, C., Pols, J., Domenech, M., Moser, I. and EFORTT Investigators (2015) Ethical implications of home telecare for older people: a framework derived from a multisited participative study. *Health Expectations: An International Journal of Public Participation in Health Care and Health Policy* 18(3): 438–49.

Mort, M., Roberts, C.M., Furbo, M.K., Wilkinson, J. and Mackenzie, A. (2016) Biosensing: how citizens' views illuminate emerging health and social risks. *Health, Risk and Society* 17(7/8): 605–23.

Murphy, M. (2012) *Seizing the means of reproduction: Entanglements of feminism, health, and technoscience*. Durham, NC: Duke University Press.

Nafus, D. (2013) The data economy of biosensors. In: McGrath, M., Ni Scanaill, C., and Nafus, D. (eds) *Sensor technologies: Healthcare, wellness and environmental applications*. New York: Apress Open.

Nafus, D. (2016a) Introduction. In: Nafus, D. (ed) *Quantified: Biosensing technologies in everyday life* (1st edn). Cambridge, MA: MIT Press, pp ix-xxxi.

Nafus, D. (2016b) *Quantified: Biosensing technologies in everyday life*. Cambridge, MA: MIT Press, pp 137-56.

Natural Cycles (2018) Quality assured & recognised – contraception – natural cycles. Available at: www.naturalcycles.com/en/science/ certifications (accessed 9 November 2018).

Neff, G. and Nafus, D. (2016) *Self tracking*. Cambridge, MA: MIT Press.

NHS (National Health Service) (2013) NHS England sets out the next steps of public awareness about care.data. Available at: www. england.nhs.uk/2013/10/care-data/ (accessed 8 May 2018).

Nissenbaum, H. and Patterson H. (2016) Biosensing in context: health privacy in a connected world, In: Nafus, D. (ed) *Quantified: Biosensing technologies in everyday life* (1st edn). Cambridge, MA: MIT Press, pp 79-100.

Northshire (2018) Call data provided to Atkinson by Northshire's service provider. Personal communication.

Ombelet, W., Cooke, I., Dyer, S., Serour, G. and Devroey, P. (2008). Infertilty and the provision of infertility medical services in developing countries. *Human Reproduction Update* 14(6): 605-621

Oudshoorn, N. (2003) *The male pill: A biography of a technology in the making.* Durham, NC: Duke University Press.

Oxlund, B. and Whyte, S.R. (2014) Measuring and managing bodies in the later life course. *Journal of Population Ageing; Dordrecht* 7(3): 217–30.

Pannurat, N., Thiemjarus, S. and Nantajeewarawat, E. (2014) Automatic fall monitoring: a review. *Sensors (Basel, Switzerland)* 14(7): 12900–36.

Panofsky, A. (2015) From behavior genetics to postgenomics. In: Stevens, H. and Richardson, S. (eds) *Postgenomics: Perspectives on biology after the genome.* Durham, NC: Duke University Press, pp 150–73.

Pantzar, M. and Ruckenstein, M. (2017) Living the metrics: self-tracking and situated objectivity. *Digital Health* 3: 1-10.

Pantzar, M., Ruckenstein, M. and Mustonen, V. (2017) Social rhythms of the heart. *Health Sociology Review* 26(1): 22–37.

Patmore, A. (2006) *The truth about stress.* London: Atlantic Books.

Peace-Brewer, A.L. (2009) *Smart nutrition adrenal stress test sample report.* Available at: https://smartnutrition.co.uk/wp-content/uploads/2009/07/Smart-Nutrition-Adrenal-Stress-Test-Sample-Report.pdf (accessed 4 May 2018).

Petersen, A. (2015) *Hope in health: The socio-politics of optimism.* Basingstoke: Palgrave Macmillan.

Philips (2018) eCAC program: Telehealth program for chronic ambulatory care. Available at: www.philips.co.uk/healthcare/product/HCNOCTN509/ecac-program-telehealth-program-for-chronic-ambulatory-care (accessed 7 November 2018).

Pickard, S. (2009) Governing old age: the 'case managed' older person. *Sociology: The Journal of the British Sociological Association* 43(1): 67–84.

Pickard, S. (2011) Health, illness and normality: the case of old age. *BioSocieties* 6(3): 323–41.

Plantin, J.-C., Lagoze, C., Edwards, P.N. and Sandvig, C. (2016) Infrastructure studies meet platform studies in the age of Google and Facebook. *New Media & Society* 20(1): 293-310.

Pogue, D. (2018) Fitbit heart data reveals its secrets. Video, *Yahoo Finance*, 27 August. Available at: https://finance.yahoo.com/news/exclusive-fitbits-150-billion-hours-heart-data-reveals-secrets-human-health-133124215.html (accessed 14 September 2018).

Pols, J. (2012) *Care at a distance: On the closeness of technology.* Amsterdam: Amsterdam University Press.

Porges, S.W. (2011) *The polyvagal theory: Neurophysiological foundations of emotions, attachment, communication, and self-regulation (Norton series on interpersonal neurobiology).* New York: W.W. Norton & Company.

Pritchard, H., Gabrys, J. and Houston, L. (2018) Re-calibrating DIY: testing digital participation across dust sensors, fry pans and environmental pollution. *New Media & Society* 20(12): 4533–52.

Purvis, K.B., Cross, D.R. and Sunshine, W.L. (2007) *The connected child.* New York, NY: McGraw-Hill.

Pym, H. (2014) NHS plans 'kitemark' for health apps. *BBC News*, 13 November. Available at: www.bbc.com/news/health-30027504 (accessed 15 November 2018).

Rabeharisoa, V., Moreira, T. and Akrich, M. (2014) Evidence-based activism: patients' organisations, users' and activist's groups in knowledge. *BioSocieties* 9: 111–28.

Radnor, A. (2017) 'We're having a menstrual liberation': how periods got woke. *The Guardian*, 11 November. Available at: www.theguardian.com/society/2017/nov/11/periods-menstruation-liberation-women-activists-abigail-radnor (accessed 24 November 2018).

Regalado, A. (2018) 2017 was the year consumer DNA testing blew up. *MIT Technology Review*, 12 February. Available at: www.technologyreview.com/s/610233/2017-was-the-year-consumer-dna-testing-blew-up/ (accessed 10 October 2018).

Rettberg, J.W. (2014) *Seeing ourselves through technology: How we use selfies, blogs and wearable devices to see and shape ourselves.* New York, NY: Palgrave Macmillan.

Richards, M. (2010) Reading the runes of my genome: a personal exploration of retail genetics. *New Genetics and Society* 29(3): 291–310.

Richardson, S.S. and Stevens, H. (2015) *Postgenomics: Perspectives on biology after the genome*. Durham, NC: Duke University Press.

Roberts, C. (2007) *Messengers of sex: Hormones, biomedicine and feminism*. Cambridge: Cambridge University Press.

Roberts, C. (2015) Psychology, evolution and the traumatised child: exploring the neurophysiology of early sexual development. *Australian Feminist Studies* 30(86): 377–85.

Roberts, C. (2016) Tanner's puberty scale: exploring the historical entanglements of children, scientific photography and sex. *Sexualities* 19(3): 328–46.

Roberts, C. and Franklin, S. (2004) Experiencing new forms of genetic choice: findings from an ethnographic study of preimplantation genetic diagnosis. *Human Fertility* 7(4): 285–93.

Roberts, C., Mort, M. and Milligan, C. (2012) Calling for care: 'disembodied' work, teleoperators and older people living at home. *Sociology* 46(3): 490–506.

Roof, J. (2007) *The poetics of DNA*. Minneapolis, MN: University of Minnesota Press.

Rose, N. (2007) *The politics of life itself: Biomedicine, power, and subjectivity in the twenty-first century*. Princeton, NJ: Princeton University Press.

Rose, N. (2013) The human sciences in a biological age. *Theory, Culture & Society* 30(1): 3–34.

Rose, N. and Abi-Rached, J.M. (2013) *Neuro – The new brain sciences and the management of the mind*. Princeton, NJ, and Oxford: Princeton University Press.

Sanders, R. (2017) Self-tracking in the digital era: biopower, patriarchy, and the new biometric body projects. *Body & Society* 23(1): 36–63.

Saukko, P. (2009) Genetic risk online and offline: two ways of being susceptible to blood clots. *Health Risk & Society* 11(1): 1–16.

Scherwitzl, E.B., Hirschberg, A.L. and Scherwitzl, R. (2015) Identification and prediction of the fertile window using NaturalCycles. *The European Journal of Contraception & Reproductive Health Care* 20(5): 403–8.

Setton, R., Tierney, C. and Tsai, T. (2016) The accuracy of web sites and cellular phone applications in predicting the fertile window. *Obstetrics and Gynecology* 128(1): 58–63.

Sharon, T. (2018) Let's move beyond critique – but please, let's not depoliticize the debate. *The American Journal of Bioethics* 18(2): 20–2.

Smart Nutrition (2018) Adrenal stress test. *Smart Nutrition*. Available at: https://smartnutrition.co.uk/health-tests/adrenal-stress-test/ (accessed 7 November 2018).

Srnicek, N. (2016) *Platform capitalism*. New York: John Wiley & Sons.

Stacey, J. (2000) The global within: consuming nature, embodying health. In: Franklin, S., Lury, C. and Stacey, J. (eds) *Global nature, global culture*. London: Sage, pp 97–145.

Stevens, H. (2011) On the means of bio-production: bioinformatics and how to make knowledge in a high-throughput genomics laboratory. *Biosocieties* 6(2): 217–42.

Steventon, A., Bardsley, M., Billings, J., Dixon, J., Doll, H., Beynon, M., Hirani, S., Cartwright, M., Rixon, L., Knapp, M., Henderson, C., Rogers, A., Hendy, J., Fitzpatrick, R. and Newman, S. (2013) Effect of telecare on use of health and social care services: findings from the Whole Systems Demonstrator cluster randomised trial. *Age and Ageing* 42(4): 501–8.

Suchman, L. (2002) Located accountabilities in technology production. *Scandinavian Journal of Information Systems* 14(2): 91–105.

Suchman, L. (2012) Configuration. In: Lury, C. and Wakeford, N. (eds) *Inventive methods: The happening of the social*. New York, NY, and London: Routledge.

Sunder Rajan, K. (2006) *Biocapital: The constitution of postgenomic life*. Durham, NC: Duke University Press.

Throsby, K. (2004) *When IVF fails: Feminism, infertility and the negotiation of normality*. Basingstoke: Palgrave Macmillan.

Throsby, K. and Roberts, C. (2010) Getting bigger: children's bodies, genes and environments. *The Sociological Review* 58(1): 73–92.

Tin, I. (2018) The journey of a single data point. What happens when you track your cycle. 19 September. Available at: https://helloclue.com/articles/about-clue/the-journey-of-a-single-data-point (accessed 3 November 2018).

Tironi, M. and Rodríguez Giralt, I. (2017) Healing, knowing, enduring: care and politics in damaged worlds. *The Sociological Review* 65(2): 89–109.

Torous, J. and Roberts, L.W. (2017) Needed innovation in digital health and smartphone applications for mental health: transparency and trust. *JAMA Psychiatry* 74(5): 437–8.

Tucker, I. and Goodings, L. (2015) Managing stress through the Stress Free app: practices of self-care in digitally mediated spaces. *Digital Health* 1: 1–10.

Tunstall (2018a) Tunstall Vibby – fall detector. *Tunstall*. Available at: https://uk.tunstall.com/services/our-products/vibby/ (accessed 12 November 2018).

Tunstall (2018b) Solutions for social care – connected care technology. *Tunstall*. Available at: https://uk.tunstall.com/solutions-social-care/ (accessed 30 November 2018).

Tunstall Group Ltd (2014) iVi™ 'the intelligent pendant' with auto fall detection. Programming and installation guide. Available at: http://apac.tunstall.com/Uploads/Documents/iVi_intelligent_pendant_Programming_Guide_V4.pdf (accessed 22 June 2018).

Tutton, R. (2016) *Genomics and the reimagining of personalized medicine.* New York, NY and London: Routledge.

US National Library of Medicine, G.H. (2018) What are single nucleotide polymorphisms (SNPs)? *Genetics Home Reference.* Available at: https://ghr.nlm.nih.gov/primer/genomicresearch/snp (accessed 21 February 2018).

Van Andel, H.W.H., Jansen, L.M.C., Grietens, H., Knorth, E.J. and Van der Gaag, R.J. (2014) Salivary cortisol: a possible biomarker in evaluating stress and effects of interventions in young foster children? *European Child & Adolescent Psychiatry* 23(1): 3–12.

Waldby, C. and Cooper, M. (2010) From reproductive work to regenerative labour: the female body and the stem cell industries. *Feminist Theory* 11(1): 3–22.

Weaver, M. (2018) Watchdog calls for warnings on DNA testing sites. *The Guardian*, 18 September. Available at: https://www.theguardian.com/society/2018/sep/18/watchdog-calls-for-warnings-on-dna-testing-sites

Weigel, M. (2016) 'Fitbit for your period': the rise of fertility tracking. *The Guardian*, 23 March. Available at: https://www.theguardian.com/technology/2016/mar/23/fitbit-for-your-period-the-rise-of-fertility-tracking

West, P., Van Kleek, M., Giordano, R., Weal, M. and Shadbolt, N. (2017) Information quality challenges of patient-generated data in clinical practice. *Frontiers in Public Health* 5, 284. doi: 10.3389/fpubh.2017.00284

WHO (World Health Organisation) (2006) *Constitution of the World Health Organization – Basic Documents* (45th edn, supplement). Available at: https://www.who.int/governance/eb/who_constitution_en.pdf

WHO (World Health Organisation) (2018) Global prevalence of infertility, infecundity and childlessness. Available at: www.who.int/reproductivehealth/topics/infertility/burden/en/ (accessed 10 November 2018).

Wikipedia (2017) Nanotechnology/biosensors – Wikibooks, open books for an open world. 25 November. Available at: https://en.wikibooks.org/wiki/Nanotechnology/Biosensors (accessed 29 November 2018).

Wilkinson, J. (2014) Unpublished PhD data.

Wilkinson, J. (2016) *Ovulation biosensors: Emerging practices of knowing and sensing*. Unpublished PhD thesis. Lancaster: Lancaster University.

Wilkinson, J., Roberts, C. and Mort, M. (2015) Ovulation monitoring and reproductive heterosex: living the conceptive imperative? *Culture, Health & Sexuality* 17(4): 454–69.

Wilson, C.N. (2018) Let's talk about periods! 11 February. Available at: www.youtube.com/watch?v=LWA53LU4xcI (accessed 10 November 2018).

Wise, J. (2016) Activity trackers, even with cash incentives, do not improve health. *BMJ* 355: i5392.

Woolham, J.G., Steils, N., Fisk, M., Porteus, J. and Forsyth, K. (2018) The UTOPIA project. *Using telecare for older people in adult social care: the findings of a 2016–17 national survey of local authority telecare provision for older people in England.* Social Care Workforce Research Unit, King's College London. Available at: https://kclpure.kcl.ac.uk/portal/files/87498580/Utopia_project_report.pdf

Zeiler, K. and Malmquist, A. (2014) Lesbian shared biological motherhood: the ethics of IVF with reception of oocytes from partner. *Medicine, Health Care and Philosophy* 17(3): 347–55.

Index